Sexuality and Disability

Maddie Blackburn
RGN RM Higher Dip HV Cert HEd MSc Grad Dip Law
Grad Dip Legal Practice

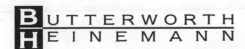

OXFORD AUCKLAND BOSTON JOHANNESBURG MELBOURNE NEW DELHI

Butterworth-Heinemann
An imprint of Elsevier
Linacre House, Jordan Hill, Oxford OX2 8DP
225 Wildwood Avenue, Woburn, MA 01801-2041

First published 2002

British Library Cataloguing in Publication Data
Blackburn, Maddie
  Sexuality and disability
  1. Disabled – Sexual behaviour
  I. Title
  362.4

ISBN 0 7506 2252 0

1003127114

Typeset by Avocet Typeset, Brill, Aylesbury, Bucks
Printed and bound in Great Britain by Biddles Ltd, Guildford and Kings Lynn

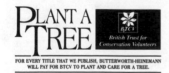

Contents

Acknowledgements

I am grateful for the advice, support and encouragement of many individuals and organizations. I am indebted to the Association for Spina Bifida and/or Hydrocephalus (ASBAH) for awarding a Research Fellowship that enabled the work to be carried out.

Most of all, I am grateful to all the young people who gave generously of their time and allowed me into the privacy of their lives, to discuss both personal and intimate experiences. This text has taken some time to conclude as I decided to retrain as a lawyer in search of some of the answers that I was unable to find or answer at the time this work was undertaken. Despite retraining, some of the questions still remain difficult to answer but offered me further insight into the rights of disabled people!

Particular thanks are extended to Dr Martin Bax, Senior Research Fellow; Imogen Carlton; D.J.R. Morgan, Senior Lecturer in Therapeutics; Imperial College Medical School, London, formerly Charing Cross and Westminster Medical Schools, London; The Social Policy Research Unit, University of York; Daman Bahl and Sue Simmonds. Members of the advisory panel at the time of the research: Mr Alan I. Hannah; Mrs Pat Edser; Mr John Naudé; Ms Heather Nicholas; Dr David Grant; Ms Yvonne Hunt; Mr Brian Walsh; Mr Julian Shah; Leonie Holgate; Mary White; Simon Coote. And finally: Mario, Tommaso, Laura Impallomeni and Daniel Wilson, my faithful computer, espresso coffee, and Classic FM!

Dedications

For those who care to care for care....

In memory of the late Professor Ann Craft and Paul Toothill, who provided much inspiration for this work.

Preface

'Sex ... Is this something *only* to talk about ... particularly if you are a disabled person ... or is it something that regardless of a disability ... everyone can enjoy too'. This was just one of many comments raised by disabled people who took part in this particular research. This book focuses on research undertaken by myself, at the time of undertaking this research I was a specialist health visitor[1] working with Dr Martin Bax, a paediatrician who supervised this research. The text aims to explore some of the issues raised by the first question while providing guidance for multi-disciplinary professionals who work primarily with physically disabled young[2] adults. The research raised many issues about sex, education and relationships for disabled people, which are addressed. Throughout the research, which involved interviews with both disabled and able-bodied young people, I soon realized that the level of sexual knowledge as well as relationship experiences varied for many young disabled people. Most of the young people I interviewed had spina bifida, either with or without hydrocephalus. I also spoke to non-disabled people about their sexuality, although their views are not discussed in detail here. There are other detailed texts that address the sexuality of able-bodied people (see Bibliography and Useful Organizations and Addresses). After the research was completed, the disabled young people requested that information about sex should be produced in a format that would help both professional staff as well as themselves. In addition, young people were concerned that this work should not end up solely as a report from which only academics would benefit! The end product was not only a book but training materials, produced by Martin and myself in collaboration with other specialists (see Acknowledgements). The materials include *Sexuality and Disability in Spina Bifida and Hydrocephalus*[3], *You, Your Partner and Continence – an Introduction to Sexuality, Disability and Continence*[4] and *Peter's Story – the Cost of*

---

[1] I am now a solicitor, specializing in health care, with an emphasis on children's issues.
[2] Some adults may also have learning difficulties.
[3] In conjunction with Dr Martin Bax and the former Charing Cross and Westminster Medical School Television Unit.
[4] Produced by Imogen Carlton and the Thames Valley University, Media and Cultural Sciences Unit in collaboration with the former Charing Cross and Westminster Medical School and ASBAH.

Incontinence[5], the latter which was produced with an award by the Royal College of Nursing and Gulbenkian Foundation. *Peter's Story* was submitted for a best script award to the Prix Leonardo Medical Education awards, Parma, Italy in 1995. It also received a Bronze Certificate of Education Merit by the British Medical Association in 1996. Since this time, the video has been screened at various national and international health care conferences.

Maddie Blackburn

---

[5] From an original case history written by Mary White. Video rewritten and produced by Mary White, Maddie Blackburn and Brian Walsh in conjunction with 'Peter' and the former Charing Cross and Westminster Medical School Television Unit at Charing Cross Hospital.

Introduction

What this text is ... and what it is not

This handbook focuses primarily on the sexual knowledge and experiences of 100 young adults, specifically with spina bifida and/or hydrocephalus. Other disabilities are briefly considered. Some comparison is made with able-bodied people, although this is not the focus of this text. Spina bifida and hydrocephalus are complex physical disabilities, which are frequently associated with some physical, neurological, sensory, urological and sometimes cognitive difficulties. It is hoped that some of the information related to people with spina bifida may help staff who work with other disabled people. It is also hoped that the text will be of interest to health care specialists, in particular rehabilitation specialists, sexual health counsellors, continence nurses, other nurses who work with disabled people, such as health visitors, district nurses and practice nurses, general practitioners, paediatricians and other medical specialists such as neurologists and urologists. However, the scope of this short handbook cannot possibly cover all aspects of Sexuality and Disability nor meet the needs of all health care specialists. I suggest that this text may be used in conjunction with or as a backup to other sexuality texts (see Bibliography). It may be read independently by specialists who work specifically with people with spina bifida and/or hydrocephalus. Although gay and lesbian relationships, cultural and religious aspects as well as HIV and AIDS are acknowledged, they are not discussed in detail within this text. Clearly there are other substantive texts specifically written about these subjects. The subject of Sexuality and Disability can sometimes be perceived as contentious. The sexuality of a disabled person should be a basic human right. Yet society often regards the sexuality of disabled people as taboo. Sexuality and Disability may become a legal nightmare in areas where arguably the law should not interfere, i.e. the feelings, instincts and emotions of disabled adults. Balancing the sexual rights of disabled people, whilst protecting disabled people who may be vulnerable and exposed to sexual exploitation, are areas where health as well as legal professionals and policy advisers often still grapple!

Terminology

I have sought to avoid pejorative language. Some seemingly gratuitous terms may be used to illustrate points but are not intended to offend any individual or groups of people. Generally, such terms are quoted from referenced literature or legislation. There has been considerable debate about acceptable definitions of 'disability' (Oliver 1990). The terms 'disabled people', 'people with disabilities', 'disabled and non-disabled person' are used interchangeably. At times, it is necessary to differentiate between people with 'learning difficulties' or 'cognitive deficits' and those with 'physical disabilities'.

1 Why sexuality and disability research?

Introducing the sexuality acronym

Sex is the most important bodily function for the preservation and propagation of the human species. However, sex is still regarded as one of the great taboos of modern society, a subject regarded by some as not to be talked about, at any time, in any place and least of all among disabled people[1]. Until recently, this trend was even more pronounced with regard to young disabled people. The international literature on this topic has been carefully reviewed in recent years (Blackburn 1993). This has confirmed the yawning gaps that exist with regard to society's understanding and perceptions about the sexual wishes of disabled people.

Sexuality: the acronym

I have used an acronym – sexuality – as an outline for the book. Each letter signifies the themes or chapters that are covered. As previously stated, the work is based on research carried out by myself and supervised by Martin Bax in the 1990s. The intention is to describe the research in a practical way so that the evidence may be applied to the health care practitioner's work. The nine letters, each signifying different aspects of sexuality, indicate the main requests, concerns and findings expressed by the disabled people who took part in the research.

Sex – the meaning of it
Differentiating between the meanings of sex, sexuality and sexual health may, at times, be confusing. Health professionals are apt to use the terms interchangeably and sometimes inappropriately. Although Appendix 5 provides young people's views and definitions of love, friendship, sex and relationships, some recognized definitions of each are included. The *Oxford Dictionary* defines sex as '…male or female; females or males collectively: sexual instinct desire or activity etc., sexual intercourse, having a specified sexual appetite…'. Sex may therefore refer to gender

---

[1] Quote from a young person in this study.

differences, as well as sexual intercourse or the desire for sexual intercourse. In contrast, sexuality is characterized and distinguished by sex, concerned with sex and the sexual characteristics of potency. Sexuality does not solely relate to sexual activity. In other words, sexuality is not just a desire for, or the act of, penetrative sex but an individual's sexual identity.

Sexuality has been described as

> An individual's self concept, shaped by their personality and expressed as sexual feelings, attitudes, beliefs and behaviours, expressed through a heterosexual, bisexual or transsexual orientation[2].

Sexual health can be described as

> The physical, emotional, psychological, social and cultural well-being of a person's identity and the capacity and freedom to enjoy and express sexuality without exploitation, oppression, physical or emotional harm.

Sexual health may either be a primary or secondary focus of care, depending on the patient's care needs. This is more apparent for some people who may need specific care to develop and promote sexual health (RCN 2000).

Education
Our first intention was to ascertain what, if any, sex education had been provided either in school, college or any other environment for young disabled people. Secondly, which groups of people were mainly responsible for providing sex education: parents, teachers, counsellors, etc.? Finally, were classroom sex education programmes the only teaching methods 'on offer'? Although Chapter 5 describes the provision and types of sex education, it is important to acknowledge at the outset that 80% of the young people interviewed had received some sex education, albeit at different stages of their school life or after leaving school or college. These young people were less concerned about the lack of sex education provision, but more concerned about the design and appropriateness of sex education available for disabled people.

'Xperiences
This research, in common with other studies, often raised further questions; for example, issues of sexual abuse and exploitation. It was not in the original research design to detail information about sexual or physical abuse. However, as some young people volunteered and raised concerns about abuse, the information from the qualitative interviews are reported here. In addition, the following were discussed. Is the disabled person's relationship experience (whether sexual or platonic) any different from

---

[2] Royal College of Nursing (2000) *Sexual Health And Nursing Practice*, adapted with permission from the Family Planning Association, publication code 000965.

their able-bodied peers? If so, do young disabled people have the same opportunity to have 'sex' as able-bodied people? Are physical relationships inhibited by physical, sensory or cognitive impairment? These important questions are addressed in Chapter 5, although providing precise answers proved difficult.

Understanding

Many young people interviewed had hydrocephalus as well as spina bifida. The former condition may impair memory and the ability to recall information. For this reason, Chapter 3 describes the complexities of both spina bifida and/or hydrocephalus, with a particular focus on cognition, drawing on the empirical literature in this field. A psychologist, Heather Nicholas, assisted us with some of the tests to assess cognition. She advised on some of the specific issues that may impair memory in this population. The psychology tests are referred to in Chapters 3–5.

Attitudes

Throughout, the young people commented on society's negative attitudes and feelings about the sexuality of disabled people. How one changes society's attitudes, without denying a disabled person the right to information and a sexually fulfilling relationship, are themes that are also considered.

Law

The Disability Discrimination Act (1995) was enforced in 1996. Although this law has increased the disabled person's rights to education, employment and access to buildings, it does not address the sexual rights of disabled people and particularly those who may require protection from sexual violation. At the time of writing, the Disability Discrimination Act was being amended. The Human Rights Act 1998 may begin to challenge the sexual rights of disabled people. Chapter 5 highlights the vulnerability of some disabled people who reported physical and sexual abuse, while Chapter 6 and Appendix 6 outline some of the laws and cases related to sexuality and disability. The law for the most part relates to the English and Welsh legal system.

Information

The young people were very explicit about how they wanted to receive information about sex. Chapter 5 provides suggestions on how disabled people would like to receive such information. Chapter 7 describes some of the training materials that have been produced since completing the research. Many young disabled people either assisted with the production of these materials or critically reviewed them.

Terminology

During the interviews, discrepancies between the young person's understanding of specific words or phrases were noted. For example, some disabled people stated that they knew the meaning of the word 'wet dream'. Many stated that they had heard the term but in reality fewer understood the precise meaning. Terms and terminology are addressed in Chapters 5 and 6.

Young adults with disabilities

Throughout, I was conscious that I was exploring the sexual needs, knowledge and information of young disabled people. Although this handbook aims to assist professionals in their work with disabled people, I acknowledge that the work has mainly been produced by an able-bodied health professional. I wish to reassure readers that disabled people were consulted for their opinions at every stage of the project. I sincerely hope that the handbook provides and reflects an accurate interpretation of their views.

The dilemmas of undertaking sexuality research

2

This work highlighted so many ethical issues that were tangential to the main research, I felt an extra chapter should be included to discuss some of the specific ethical issues that arose and may help other nurses or doctors planning to undertake sexuality research in future. However naïve it may sound, I firmly believe that some of the dilemmas that I encountered were because the word *Sex* was included in the research title. It is possible that if the study title had excluded the word *sex* or *sexuality*, then some, if not all, ethics committees might have viewed the proposal differently. This is not to infer that such committees would have been justified in scrutinizing this project less vigilantly; nor that, as research, it would have been fair in providing either a 'watered down' or less controversial title for the proposal! This was *certainly not* the objective.

Without appearing to change the emphasis of the study, suppose the research had been entitled: *The physical and emotional needs of 100 young adults with spina bifida and/or hydrocephalus* or *Knowledge and relationship experiences in a group of young adults with neural tube defects aged 16–25 years.* Would the response to this research proposal from ethics committees have differed? Arguably these titles imply the same meaning – bar using the word *sex.* Would as many ethics committees still have requested to meet the principal researcher (myself), or requested me to present the proposal to their committee(s)?

In Chapter 1, I acknowledge that sex is still regarded as a *taboo* subject for many people – not least for *some* health and legal specialists who may serve on research ethics committees. Understandably the ethics committees needed to enquire how deeply I would probe into the intimate details of people's lives.

Ethics committees – and sexuality research

When the work began, the *Sexuality and Disability* research proposal had been approved by Local Research Ethics Committees in six districts in Kent and in eleven out of twelve districts in the North West Thames Region. However, it took several months for other ethics committees to reach their decisions. Furthermore, a total of twenty-three committees were obliged to scrutinize the proposal before I could begin the main study. Understandably the research committees needed to be confident that:

- all the disabled people would be able to respond to such an interview situation, as proposed
- It was appropriate and ethical to conduct this type of research with disabled people.

I accept that these are perfectly reasonable and justified concerns for any research ethics committee to examine where the words 'sex' or 'sexuality' appear in the title. James and Platzer (1999) noted that it is rare to 'find honest accounts of the difficulties and dilemmas encountered when sensitive research is conducted with vulnerable populations'. In their work, they highlighted the difficulties for both the researchers and the needs of the gay and lesbian populations they were investigating and identified the need for support structures for both groups when undertaking such research.

The role of ethics committees – a public watchdog?

Reports and circulars have recommended that all general practitioner, dental, hospital and academic research proposals are considered by the local research ethics committee: The principle role of the Ethics Committee is that of '*a public watchdog*' whose aims are:

- to safeguard and protect the interests of the general public, in particular
- those with learning difficulties or mental impairment; and
- children under the age of consent, the elderly and the frail.

Such committees ensure that research participants are fully informed of objectives, can give informed consent, and that they have the right to withdraw from studies at any stage without fear of retribution.

Most research ethics committees require submission of a written proposal prior to approving the research. This should include: the aims; names of the key researchers; the expectations of contributors; duration and nature of the investigation; and draft consent forms. Committees will normally request a final report on completion of the study. Often committees invite the principal researcher to present, discuss and if necessary defend the research protocol with its members. Any amendments to the research made during the course of investigation should be notified in writing to the chairperson of the committee.

A case for standardization

This study necessitated the recruitment of over a 100 young adults with spina bifida and/or hydrocephalus and an equivalent number of able-bodied volunteers who agreed to provide control data (not discussed in detail here). The interviews took place in two regions but, as previously stated, required the approval of twenty-three individual ethics committees. This is despite the fact that there were only a few participants from each district. Over a third of the committees requested my presence to discuss the protocol. In some cases, this necessitated travelling long distances and waiting several hours to defend the proposal. One meeting was inquorate and therefore I was asked to return on another day. Committee recommendations often varied. Some members were concerned about inviting the participation of adults with 'learning difficulties'.

The Research Ethics Committees made the following recommendations:

- Additional verbal explanation as well as written consent prior to proceeding to the second part of the interview (see Appendix 1).
- A contact telephone number and address for disabled adults who may wish to obtain further information following interview.
- Participation of local paediatricians (one district only).
- Amendments to the letters of consent.
- A list of the numbers of people from each district who had participated.
- Consideration to using a male interviewer (not obligatory).
- Consideration to using a disabled interviewer (not obligatory).
- A report outlining major recommendations.

The Royal College of Physicians[1] have now reviewed their guidelines for multi-centred research projects. Research involving people from several areas may now be submitted and approved centrally but local research ethics committees need to retain a copy of the proposal, may elect to discuss the proposal and should be advised of any changes made.

The Researcher's responsibilities

Clearly, all health professionals have professional duties and responsibilities, primarily to their patients and clients but also to ethics committee and those funding the research. In the light of these disparate and competing responsibilities, it is important to consider for whom the research is intended:

- The funding body, in this case a charity, who may wish to use the information to develop or review current service provision?
- The researcher, in pursuit of professional development, seeking an ethical research project to gain postgraduate qualifications or publications?
- The employing body who may audit the number of research publications as well as the service provision for its patients/clients?
- The Medical Ethics Committee who may approve or reject the research proposals?
- Most of all … the disabled person who provides the evidence on which to prove or refute the researcher's original hypothesis?

---

[1] Royal College of Physicians, www.rcplondon.co.uk

If Ethical Science seeks to improve the health of the human race, then by right the information belongs to everyone and should be accessible to all the groups listed above. However, surely one should first acknowledge those people who provided the data and information, and secondly the funding body for financing the project.

Research dissemination

Nurses, doctors and in particular health researchers, are often criticized for using 'jargon' or terminology which service users do not understand. It is therefore important that information is disseminated in a language which will be appropriate to the client, the funding body and/or employer. Naturally, the language used will depend on the recipient or reader. A person with minor learning disabilities may prefer to receive information in the form of simple, pictorial leaflets, whereas a charity whose members include mainly lay members of staff, may prefer to receive information using plain English. All too frequently, the people who provide information are the last to have access or to benefit from it. Often reports are written in a style which may be difficult for those with learning difficulties, or no health care training, to interpret. Clearly, the introduction of Clinical Governance arrangements within the NHS has increased the need to include and recognize the involvement of service users, particularly those involved in research initiatives.

The funding body

The researcher should consider the following issues related to funding bodies:

- Try to complete the survey within reasonable time. Should this be difficult, state the intention to delay completion, in writing.
- Additional funding requests should be made in writing and in advance of the proposed completion date. If these are refused, draw up a list of realistic, attainable goals to be completed within a defined timescale.
- Many charities request written reports of progress. This gives some idea of the level of activity, provides an update and acknowledges the contribution of fund-raisers.
- On completion, write a precise account of findings and recommendations. If the researcher intends to use information for either private study or teaching purposes, then permission to do so should be obtained from the client and the funding body.

Research with disabled people

Researchers who work with disabled adults may encounter moral dilemmas during their work. This was certainly my experience. While some disabled adults may be able to give informed consent, the comprehension and mental capacity of some people with learning disabilities may vary. At the same time, arbitrarily excluding people with disabilities from research initiatives may fail to obtain useful knowledge[2] (Jirovec 1989) as well as being perceived as discriminatory. The same principles should apply both when people are invited to take part in research and when obtaining consent to treatment (DoH 2001).

Moral dilemmas encountered in this research

All the young disabled people were sent an explanatory letter about this research (see Appendix 1) and offered preliminary interviews to discuss any aspect or concern they might have. Six disabled adults requested *preliminary face-to-face* interviews and ten people telephoned, requesting further information, prior to their agreement. Ten parents (this also included principal carers) also sought a preliminary discussion on the young person's behalf. Four parents/carers overall refused consent (on their son/daughter's behalf). Furthermore, some parents opened their son or daughter's mail and replied and declined the invitation, often without the young person's knowledge! This highlights several issues about the rights of carers opening another adult's mail. When asked for an explanation, many parents volunteered that the subject matter was so sensitive that they preferred to answer the correspondence and not to let their sons or daughters read it.

Informed consent

Researchers should always ensure that everyone, but particularly people with disabilities, fully understand the nature, extent and time of their expected involvement in research. These principles are no different from those applied to health professionals who seek consent to treatment from their patients. Disabled people should never feel coerced into participating in any research. Furthermore, they should be advised that they may withdraw at any time and 'particular care' should be taken to ensure that sufficient time, appropriate explanation and information is available to ensure disabled people are able to absorb what they are agreeing to take part in (GMC 1998). Before inviting the disabled person, I needed to ensure that the young person was able to give informed consent.

Competency to consent is based on three integral components: *voluntary choice, knowledge and understanding*, and *competency to decide* (Thorpe 1989). The latter feature is often the most difficult to measure. Some people with learning difficulties are capable of making decisions

---

[2] In this case I am describing nurses' knowledge.

about daily routines (such as bathing, and clean intermittent catheterization) but may have difficulty in understanding more specific details about operations, treatments and research involvement.

Professor Michael Gunn (1985) has argued "*that there is no legal decision that a person who is mentally handicapped is necessarily incapable of making treatment or care decisions*" suggesting that it would not be unjust to include some people with learning difficulties in carefully planned and well-executed research.

Measures of competence may also vary according to the institution and organization where research is being undertaken. Some institutions may use psychological testing, others educational attainment, as indicators of the young person's cognitive function. How often is decision-making left to carers or relatives, using the "*Does he take sugar?*" approach, all too often disregarding the individual feelings, contributions, requests and expectations of the disabled person. Common examples here may include: admission and discharge from hospital, respite care, returning to the community after a hospital or residential unit is closed, etc. The disabled person may be given little choice about such decisions. Such actions may be a consequence of the closure of a particular institution in the first place. Furthermore, some parents/carers may be over-protective about the disabled person taking important decisions alone. Yet the disabled person *who is competent* should have the same rights to make decisions as any other person. Once the competent person reaches 18, he or she is 'adult', and that person can take decisions on any matter. Thus from at least 18[3], parents/carers and health staff have no right to make decisions on the disabled person's behalf. Under English Law, no-one can give consent to treatment and/or examination for an adult without capacity. Parents, carers or health care staff cannot consent on behalf of an adult. However, in exceptional circumstances, such as life and death situations, it may be lawful to carry out procedures or treatment without the adult's consent.

Although changes in the Law are necessary to clarify some of the above points, self advocacy *is* increasing among disabled people. Voluntary choice and explanation should be a basic human right; whether it is the choice to wear one's own clothes in hospital or the right *to be invited* to participate in research. By the same token, the disabled person is as entitled to an explanation about the research as an able-bodied individual is[4].

Methods of explaining the research

An impartial researcher should offer a preliminary, coherent explanation

---

[3] Gillick competence is discussed in Chapter 6. The Gillick Ruling applies to young people under the age of 18.

[4] Reference Guide to Consent from Examination or Treatment (2001) Department of Health.

of research objectives. An explanatory letter, including a stamped addressed envelope inviting written consent should be sent to the disabled person. The letter should be typed in plain English, avoiding jargon. If reading the written word is difficult for the disabled person, it might be helpful to include an audiocassette copy of the explanatory letter. The disabled person must be given enough time to consider and discuss the request, before giving an informed, written or witnessed verbal decision.

People with disabilities: implications for consent

The individual, whether able-bodied or disabled, has certain rights, protected by law, which should not be infringed for the public good (Medical Research Council 1991). In relation to research, this includes the adult's freedom to give or withhold consent at his or her own discretion, as well as the right to withdraw from research projects at any time without fear of retribution or any treatment being compromised. There are many health issues confronting the young disabled person, which may prevent that individual from pursuing an active and independent life and where non-therapeutic research may or may not be perceived to be of direct benefit to that person.

People with learning difficulties: implications for research

Health professionals who work with people who have learning difficulties often have to consider whether their clients can give consent and make independent, informed decisions. Some people with learning difficulties may be able to give or withhold consent and should be encouraged to do so. Others may be unable to give informed consent. Particular attention should be exercised in selecting people with learning difficulties to participate in research (DoH 1991a, 1991b). However, mental disorder does not necessarily imply incapacity. Mental disorder is defined as *"mental illness, arrested or incomplete development of mind, psychopathic disorder and any other disorder or disability of mind and mental disorder shall be construed accordingly"* (Department of Health).

The Royal College of Physicians (1996) and Medical Research Council (1991) have both suggested that it may be ethical to undertake research with adults with learning difficulties providing it adheres to stringent measures. The research must be approved by the relevant research ethics committee and demonstrate that the research is not against their best interests (DoH 2001). The Lord Chancellor's Department (1997) in *Who decides?* reviewed the definition of capacity and examined its implications for disabled people.

Recruitment

The disabled people in this survey were recruited from charity databases and hospital records. Information regarding the young person's cognitive ability was sometimes, but not always, recorded within the notes. Certain charity databases classified people with disabilities into the following groups: those with (1) minor, (2) moderate and (3) severe learning difficulties. Many charities and organizations quite reasonably dissuaded me from writing to individuals with severe learning difficulties. Some charities offered to assist by writing to those adults with minor to moderate learning difficulties who were known to their service. Before interviews the young person's permission was obtained to access information from their records about recent psychological assessments, educational attainment and general health.

Confidentiality and the duty of care

At the time of this research, the UKCC was the regulatory body for nurses, midwives and health visitors, which has now been replaced by the Nurses, Midwives Council (NMC). The new regulatory body, the NMC, came into being in April 2002. Although the Code of Professional Conduct has been modified, it still upholds many of the principles and key areas enshrined in the former UKCC code. Almost all other UKCC publications will remain valid until further notice (NMC News, Spring 2002, Number 1). Therefore, many of the above principles still apply. Clause 10 of the UKCC (1992) *Code of Professional Conduct* states that nurses, midwives and health visitors must at all times protect *"all confidential information concerning patients and clients obtained in the course of professional practice, and make disclosures only with consent, where required, by the order of a court or where you can justify disclosure in the wider public interest"*.

There is often confusion about what is regarded as 'confidential information'. This may provoke anxiety amongst both lawyers and health care specialists. The object of confidentiality is to:

- Ensure that patients/clients will continue to share sensitive and confidential information with healthcare practitioners (where considered necessary).
- Respect the wishes of the person who imparted the confidence, on the understanding that it was entrusted to facilitate care and for no other purpose.

The nurse seeks information, with consent from the client, for a research project. The disabled person then shares sensitive, confidential information during the course of an interview. Some of the information may be irrelevant to the research but may be of considerable importance in protecting and safeguarding the interests of that particular disabled person. In this study, ten people disclosed that they had previously been physically or sexually abused. On the merits of each individual case I had to decide:

- Whether or not those individuals risked further abuse.

- What were my responsibilities in the light of such disclosure?
- Was there a "Duty of Care" to disclose this information to another agency in order to protect and safeguard the young person's interests, particularly if the disabled person was unable to prevent further abuse?
- This information was only disclosed during the research interview (I had no prior knowledge of the abuse). Therefore, should this information be passed onto anyone else? If the risk of further abuse was minimal why risk creating further anxiety? If the client was thought to still be at risk, should permission be obtained to share this information with another agency, on a need to know basis, in order to protect the young person from further harm? The Department of Health's paper "No Secrets" (2000) offers guidance for professionals who might find themselves faced by such a situation.
- I had to consider my responsibilities in the light of the circumstances of each individual case. It was difficult to apply arbitrary rules on such important matters particularly for disabled people.

Professional accountability and research

Researchers are required to bring a variety of skills to their work. They need good negotiation and communication skills in order to work competently and confidently with disabled people, members of ethics committees, and medical and paramedical colleagues.

Depending on the nature of the research, there may be a conflict of interest between the respect for the advancement and pursuit of knowledge and whether research can produce the best outcomes for the client.

Nurses are often required to assist doctors in carrying out research, which sometimes involves administering prescribed drugs or treatments. The drugs may be prescribed as part of a clinical trial intended for a cancer treatment. Benjamin and Curtis (1981) described the ambivalence which some nurses felt; they supported the pursuit for cancer treatment but questioned the benefits of such experimentation on humans.

Furthermore, nurses may question their responsibilities when asked by medical colleagues to administer treatments or medications to patients on their behalf. They may feel that the particular doctor should administer these. I saw my primary task as collecting, analysing, preparing and disseminating the research in a form acceptable to both the client and the funding body. I recognized that certain duties which, if undertaken by me, would breach my professional code of practice. On such occasions, it would be my responsibility to acknowledge these boundaries and seek the assistance of others more suitably qualified to undertake such tasks. The answer for other nurse researchers, who may find such decisions difficult, is enshrined in Clause 4 of the former UKCC's (1992) *Code of Professional Conduct*. This emphasizes that nurses should "*acknowledge any limitations in your knowledge and competence and decline any duties or responsibilities unless able to perform them in a safe and skilled manner*".

Clause 6 of the former UKCC's *Code of Professional Conduct* unequivocally states that nurses and midwives should *"work in a collaborative and co-operative manner with health care professionals and others involved in providing care, and recognize and respect their particular contributions within the care team"*.

Although Alderson (1992) argued that research may not always be of mutual benefit, she hoped that research would lead to the improvement of services for those people providing the research information and in particular those with disabilities. She felt that this was extremely relevant in therapeutic research, where the research aims to be of direct benefit to the person. By contrast, non-therapeutic research is *"designed to advance scientific knowledge and therefore be of collected benefit, but not expected to give direct benefit to the research subject"* (Alderson, 1992).

Summary

Therapeutic or non-therapeutic research may help or fail to advance human knowledge (Alderson 1993). All research involving the participation of human beings must be carefully planned and well executed. Researchers, in particular, must ensure that everyone, but particularly people with physical and learning difficulties, understand the full implications and significance of their involvement so that any stress may be minimized by their participation in sexuality research. Larcher *et al.* (1997) advocated a need for multidisciplinary clinical ethics committees (CECs), which have educational, advisory and practice development roles. They suggested that such a committee could provide significant support to clinical practice. The CECs which have now been set up in the UK vary significantly in relation to their procedures, functions, structures, membership and accountability. Clearly some of the dilemmas that arose in my work might have been well-served by a clinical ethics committee had it existed at that time.

Understanding spina bifida and/or hydrocephalus – the literature, the disability

3

You may ask why people with spina bifida (SB) and hydrocephalus (HC) were selected to take part in this research. Why instead were other people with other physical disabilities, such as multiple sclerosis, or people with acquired spinal cord injuries not invited? Why was it necessary to include people who may also have a learning difficulty as well as a major physical disability? In essence, there are several reasons why the sexual knowledge and needs of people with SB and HC were chosen. Primarily, this population often have lower motor and sensory disabilities, combined with intellectual dysfunction. A hypothesis was that people with motor and sensory disabilities are more likely to experience difficulties in their physical relationships than their able-bodied peers. Furthermore, a person with a cognitive deficit is likely to have greater problems in learning and remembering information about sex, regardless of whether sex education was ever provided. Therefore, people with SB and HC often have a combination of physical and complicated neurological disabilities, worthy of investigation, particularly in relation to their sexuality. It is hoped that these findings might assist other people more widely, particularly those with complex physical sensory or neurological disabilities.

Notwithstanding, there is increasing literature addressing the medical and physical complications associated with SB (see Bannister and Tew 1991, Borzyskowski and Mundy 1990, Thomas *et al.* 1989) but only recently has attention focused on the psychological and sociological aspects of these disabilities (Appleton *et al.* 1994, Dorner 1977, 1980, 1990, Edser and Ward 1991, Tew 1991, Thomas *et al.* 1989). There is still a limited amount of literature, which examines the sexual needs of this population (Dorner 1977, Edser and Ward 1991, Sandler *et al.* 1996, Verhoef *et al.* 2000). Recent advances in medical technology mean that 90% of babies with SB/HC now survive compared with a 90% mortality rate of twenty years ago (Grenier and Cartwright 1986). Of those who survive, about 50% will live to school age (Grenier and Cartwright 1986) many of whom will reach adulthood. It is therefore understandable that information and teaching about peer and sexual relationships will be necessary for these young people. It is difficult to examine the particular information and sexual needs of people with SB/HC without first considering the specific and often complex features of these disabilities and some background is provided below.

Spina bifida and/or hydrocephalus – the facts

Hydrocephalus usually accompanies open (described later in this chapter) spina bifida. Both conditions are often described together as they share many aetiological and epidemiological features (Smithells 1991). Approximately 75% of children with SB have HC (Brocklehurst *et al.* 1976). Birth prevalence varies throughout the world, between individual ethnic and social groups and from one decade to another in particular populations (Smithells 1991). In 1980, Elwood and Elwood noted that global birth prevalence ranged from 10 to 0.1 per 1000 births. In England and Wales there has been a significant reduction in the numbers of babies born with SB/HC in the last decade (Rankin *et al.* 2000). The physiological and cognitive features of both SB and HC are addressed below.

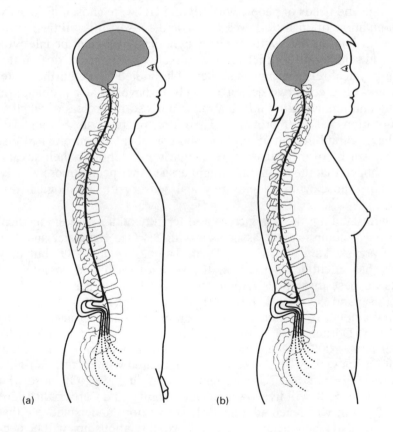

(a)   (b)

Figure 3.1   Spina bifida

Spina bifida

The recorded history of SB dates back to the eighteenth century, when *Morgagni* first described its association with HC. Lebedeff (1881) noted that SB was a failure of the neural tube to close during embryological development. More recently, Brocklehurst *et al.* (1976) described SB as a "*congenital developmental anomaly of one or more of the vertebrae and spinal processes of the spinal column effecting both limbs and neurogenic function*". The spinal vertebrae fail to form properly, leaving a split or gap (ASBAH 1991a). Since both SB and HC are complex disabilities, a brief description of the central nervous system and the spinal anatomy is provided, in an attempt to address some of the implications, when dealing with sexual matters.

The spine is made up of thirty-three bones or vertebrae, whose major function is to support muscles and to protect the spinal cord (Figure 3.2). The central nervous system is responsible for the sensory mechanisms of taste, smell, sight and touch. The spinal cord forms part of this complicated and vulnerable network and requires adequate protection. The spine, in addition to the spinal cord, forms part of the neural tube, the latter developing between the 14th and 25th day following conception. The brain and spinal cord develop from the neural tube. The neural tube

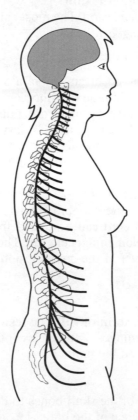

Figure 3.2   The spine

in SB fails to develop properly and becomes bifid, i.e. divided or split. The 'split' may occur in one or more vertebrae around, above or below waist level (ASBAH 1991a).

Spina bifida occulta (hidden)

In 1886, Von Recklinghausen first described spina bifida occulta as "*a symptomatic bony defect, rarely causing major disability*". The occulta is often only diagnosed in later life, in otherwise able-bodied individuals, who receive lumbar or upper sacral vertebrae X-rays for unrelated conditions. The spinal cord and meninges are rarely damaged. The occulta may be disassociated from HC. Occasionally infants are born with an epithelialized skin covering the spina bifida lesion. '*A pad of*' or an excess of hair in the lumbar-sacral region or a dermal sinus, i.e. an ectodermal abnormality, may be visible from the skin to the 'bifid' vertebra and occasionally into the dura. Brocklehurst *et al.* (1976) reported that about one in ten of the population have spina bifida occulta. For most people, its presence is of no consequence. Occasionally the spinal cord catches against the vertebrae, and becomes 'tethered'. This may subsequently affect mobility, bladder control or both.

Spina bifida aperta (open lesion)

There are two types of open lesion. The most common as well as the most serious is the *Myelomeningocele.*

Myelomeningocele

A myelomeningocele may occur anywhere along the spinal column but most commonly occurs within the mid-thoracic, lumbar and lumbosacral regions (Bannister 1991). The spinal cord fails to develop. The neural tissue and the spinal canal are exposed to injury and infection. The nerve centres controlling movement and feeling in the lower body are usually damaged, most commonly resulting in mobility difficulties, bladder and bowel incontinence (see Bannister and Tew 1991, Borzyskowski and Mundy 1990, Brocklehurst *et al.* 1976). There is often loss of sensation and some paralysis below the vertebrae, particularly within the lumbar-sacral region. The spinal cord can be traced from the upper end of the spinal canal into the myelomeningocele sac. The degree of disability will largely depend on the level of the spinal lesion, as well as the extent of nerve damage.

Meningocele

This is the least common form of SB. The lesion contains tissues which cover the spinal cord (meninges) and cerebrospinal fluid (CSF). The CSF protects the spinal cord and the brain.

Encephalocele

This is caused by failure of the skull bones to develop, resulting in some brain damage. In the absence of the brain, i.e. anencephaly, the baby will either be stillborn or die soon after birth. Rarer forms of SB, such as ventralis, hemi and true myelocele, have been described by Brocklehurst *et al.* (1976).

Aetiology of spina bifida

The precise cause of SB remains unknown, although nutritional deficiencies, in particular vitamin folates have been linked as a possible cause (Smithells 1991). The Medical Research Council Study Group (1991) reported a reduction in SB births when folate supplements were prescribed to mothers at risk. Since then, following several national campaigns, folates have been added to various cereals and foods.

Hydrocephalus

Hydrocephalus is both a congenital and/or acquired defect. It is frequently associated with open spina bifida but it is *"appropriate to consider hydrocephalus as distinct from ... spina bifida because it is known to be aetiologically heterogeneous"*. Isolated HC has more diverse origins and its epidemiology is less well-documented (Smithells 1991). Although the number of babies born with SB have declined over the last decade, the incidence of HC, resulting from intraventricular haemorrhage, has unfortunately increased, often as a result of improved survival of low birth

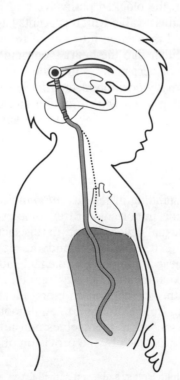

Figure 3.3 Hydrocephalus

weight babies (Forrest 1991). Some forms of paediatric HC may be associated with congenital disorders, prematurity or *Dandy-Walker Cysts* (fluid filled sacs). Hydrocephalus may also occur in adults; for example, post-haemorrhage, meningitis, tumours, etc. *Hydrocephalus is an accumulation and imbalance of the production and drainage of cerebrospinal fluid into the circulation, leading to a build-up of pressure resulting in damage to the brain tissue* (ASBAH 1991b).

Cerebrospinal fluid is produced continuously within the four ventricles of the brain. It passes through the narrow pathways, intraventricular spaces, into the brain and down the spinal cord. If the drainage pathways are blocked, the fluid accumulates in the ventricles, causing swelling and compression of the surrounding tissues. The head enlarges in babies and infants, as the skull bones are not completely fused together until the infant is approximately 18-months-old (the head size in older children and adults does not usually increase because the skull bones will have ultimately fused together). Brocklehurst *et al.* (1976) noted that over 75% of babies born with SB have HC. The complications associated with HC are varied. These include cognitive and perceptual problems, difficulties with fine movements in the hands, and clumsiness.

A major technological invention of the 1960s was the *Spitz Holter* shunt[1]. This was designed to drain off excess CSF. The valve led to a significant reduction in the number of SB related deaths. This device diverts accumulated CSF from the blocked pathways returning it to the bloodstream. The shunt contains a valve which prevents back-flow and controls drainage. The upper end is inserted into one of the ventricles, whilst the lower end is inserted either into the heart (ventriculo atrial) or abdomen (ventriculo peritoneal) or occasionally into the lungs (ventriculo pleural shunt). Shunts are normally positioned for life, but may require revision or replacement according to growth, infection and blockages. Since the Spitz Holter shunt was first devised, several different types of valves have been developed.

The literature

To gain a better understanding of the *sexual knowledge and experiences* of these young adults, it is important to offer some explanation about adolescence, growth and sexual development. In this section some of the features of socialization, experimentation and the development of social skills are discussed. These are important to enable adolescent growth and the development of sexual identity. Self-esteem and body image, as well as the development of the sexual ego and moral identity, are fundamental to the smooth transition from childhood to adulthood.

How a disabled person views themselves and how others respond to them may be influenced as much by the provision of appropriate sex edu-

---

[1] One of the inventors, Sir John Holter, had a son named Casey who ultimately died from hydrocephalus.

cation as well the disabled person's self-esteem, physical growth and development. Dorner (1977) noted that young adults with SB/HC were very interested in the opposite sex, but often had limited opportunities to meet and have relationships. His study did not specifically explore homosexual feelings and relationships.

So what about adolescence?

Surviving the teenage years or the period known as adolescence is a challenge not only for parents but for all young people, irrespective of whether they are able-bodied or disabled. Growing up and surviving adolescence may be particularly compounded by physical or learning disabilit(ies). Neinstein (1991) described three psychosocial phases of adolescence. These are as follows:

- **Stage 1** or early adolescence – this usually occurs between 11 and 14 years.
- **Stage 2** or mid-adolescence – this usually occurs between 15–18 years.
- **Stage 3** late adolescence – this usually occurs sometime between 18–21 years.

Adolescence has been studied in many areas of developmental medicine and the literature confirms that this is a period of great upheaval and change (Neinstein 1991). Anna Freud (1937, 1946) described adolescence as a period where there are alterations in drive, ego organization, object relations, and social roles. She stated that such features are characteristic of this period and will inevitably give rise to some developmental disturbances in the young person; changes and developments which will eventually lead to adult independence. The adolescent is therefore faced with the triple task of detaching his or herself from the family, discovering him or herself and learning to be accepted within a teenage society. If they are successful, hopefully s/he will be equipped for ultimate migration into the adult world! In 1963, Erikson debated the concept of a '*moratorium*' during adolescence. As he saw it, adequacy of development at one developmental stage enabled the next stage to occur, recognizing that the timing and progress of development may vary among individuals (Wilson 1998). He also recognized that any society has to give the young person some leeway for experimentation and development. This will require adults, in particular parents, to accept that adolescent experimentation is not unusual, in order for the young person to develop adult characteristics and to find out which societal niche he or she belongs to.

Self-concept and identity are important aspects of such social development. Adolescence is a period when both able-bodied and disabled people are particularly sensitive about their appearance and how others think of them (Neinstein 1991). For the able-bodied teenager social activities often increase during this period. It is a time when interpersonal and peer relationships may undergo radical changes. It is also a period when sexual awareness is heightened and the quests for independence and autonomy are increased. Belonging to a group, dating, experimenting with fashion, going to pubs, parties, 'clubbing', taking part in sports, *or engaging in behaviour such as substance, alcohol and drug misuse* may enable the young person to cope with ensuing self-image difficulties.

Almost 2500 years ago Socrates observed certain behaviour changes in adolescents:

> Our adolescents now seem to have luxury. They have bad manners and con-tempt for authority. They show disrespect for adults and spend more time hanging around places gossiping with one another ... they are ready to con-tradict their parents, monopolise the conversation in company, eat glutto-nously and tyrannise their teachers.

At a time when there appears to be increasing autonomy for able-bodied teenagers, the experiences of physically disabled adolescents may be in sharp contrast. Philip and Duckworth (1982) noted that the disabled teenager, whilst seeking to achieve independence, is expected to perform better. Sometimes the disabled person *may not* accept or recognize that he or she may be constrained by mobility difficulties, and have problems which may not be experienced by their able-bodied peers. Furthermore, Thomas *et al.* (1989) noted that disabled people experience greater hurdles in social situations than their able-bodied peers.

Undoubtedly, physical and communication difficulties may also lead to social disability. Dorner's (1977) empirical study of sixty-three adoles-cents with SB indicated an 85% incidence of depression. He noted that depressive feelings were exacerbated for both male and female groups by poor mobility, the severity of the disability and social isolation. The cor-relation between misery and social isolation was notably higher in females. Clinical evidence of emotional distress and disturbance has also been reported by Freeman (1970). Karoly (1988), looking at a *chronically ill population*, observed that this adolescent group were more susceptible to depression. He felt that this was attributable to the following: (1) gaining independence from enmeshed family systems that have not fos-tered independent functioning from the outset; and (2) joining a peer group that perceives the severely disabled child as being 'different'.

Karoly stated that the family system has a profound influence on the developing child and adolescent, particularly in relation to their physical and psychological health and sexual status: *"An enmeshed family system traps family members in an intense but stifling relationship that, while temporarily decreasing anxiety, does so by interfering with continuing maturation"* Karoly (1988).

Social skills

There have been a number of studies which have suggested that disabled children and adults are impoverished in social experience and in interper-sonal relationships (Anderson and Clark 1982, Dorner 1977). Such deprivations not only lead to difficulty in the establishment of meaningful relationships but may curtail development of social skills (Anderson and Clark 1982, Jowett 1982, Tew 1973, Thomas and Smyth 1988, Thomas *et al.* 1989). Thomas and Smyth (1988) looked at the provision of services for the disabled adult and the difficulties they encountered in skilled social behaviour. Fifty-seven young physically disabled people (mean age = 21) were compared to a group of sixty two able-bodied people (mean age = 20) using a social skills questionnaire. Thomas' results indicated that although both non-disabled and disabled people had some difficulties in most social situations, the degree of difficulty experienced by disabled people was significantly greater.

Socialization

During adolescence, there is a surge in the development of identity and recognition of the need for autonomy. It is through social interaction that the making and breaking of many relationships occur. Thomas *et al.* (1989) suggested that the sense of identity or self-image changes are in response to the differences between how people perceive themselves and how others perceive them. From about 12 years of age, the social activities of the young person increase quite substantially. Peer group activities usually begin to dominate, often with the same sex. Later, there will be more one-to-one relationships, which will become deeper, more involved and will usually, although not necessarily, include the opposite sex (if this is the person's sexual orientation). Through social activities and making friends, the teenager is able to confirm and develop his or her own personality, identity and sexuality. During this period, the adolescent's responses may be vulnerable to the reactions of those in his or her environment. Such people may include teachers, parents, carers and his or her own peer group (Anderson and Clark 1982).

It may be difficult for the able-bodied adolescent to achieve a full and satisfactory social and sex life. They must overcome many prejudices such as parental authority and disapproval, financial restrictions, educational demands, etc. before finding a compatible person or group. For the disabled teenager, these everyday problems may be further compounded by the difficulties caused by restricted mobility, incontinence, poor access facilities, illness, peer pressure and personal acceptability. The likelihood of the disabled adolescent facing increased isolation at a time when their social circle should be increasing has been frequently described (Anderson and Clark 1982, Castree and Walker 1981, Rutter *et al.* 1970, Thomas *et al.* 1989).

Self esteem

In their study of young people with cerebral palsy and spina bifida, Anderson and Clark (1982) obtained information about self-esteem and coping with new situations. In this research, both parents and young people have provided information. Parents regarded 44% of the physically disabled young people as being fearful of new situations as compared to 22% of parents of able-bodied young people. These studies highlighted issues related to the disabled person's quality of life.

Spina bifida may sometimes carry catastrophic and significant physiological and/or psychological complications (Thomas *et al*. 1989). This may well leave the young person in a state of unknowingness as to what extent, if at all, they will be able to function as ordinary social and sexual individuals. Physical disability, in addition to chronic illness and social stigma may increase social and sexual isolation. The everyday difficulties faced by the able-bodied adolescent are increased for the disabled person, for whom self-identity and the achievement of independence (within the parameters of his or her disability) are equally as important. Anderson and Spain (1977) reported:

> There is a surprising failure to recognise the acute problems of isolation from their peers that confront many of the more seriously handicapped adolescents, who face, often without the chance to satisfy them, the normal urges of young people for companionship, relations with the opposite sex, sport, enjoyment of leisure pursuits, travel, spending money, achievement, and the prospects of their own future and family.

The degree of self-satisfaction, personal fulfilment and stability any young person experiences upon reaching adulthood is frequently determined as a measure of how that individual has learnt to adapt, cope with and manage the experiences of their earlier years. Psychoanalytical theory proposes that these experiences, from birth onwards, will impact on psychological functioning in later life. However, the measure of a young person's self-esteem may also be determined in other ways. These may include positive feedback from peers and family, as well as the young person's level of social acceptance, integration, independence and autonomy permitted by the family and society. In 1981 Battle noted that:

> An individual's perception of self develops gradually and becomes more differentiated as he matures and interacts with significant others.

Body image

As far back as 1935, Schilder described body image as: "*The picture of our own body which we form in our mind, that is to say that way in which our own body appears to ourselves*". How the development of self-image, body deformity or of a distorted body image is perceived by disabled young people is now recognized (see Appleton *et al*. 1994, Offer *et al*. 1984). Irrefutably, the major biological changes that occur in a normally developing body have their affects on every young person. The adjustments that adolescents must make to a changing and maturing body will inevitably have a profound impact. Davies and Furnham (1986) examined body satisfaction in female adolescents and noted a definite decline in satisfaction over time. Older adolescents expressed particular dissatisfaction with their waist and hips. It has been suggested that these features, connected most closely to sexual identification, are those which cause maximum concern. Lerner and Karabenik (1974) found that females view their bodies primarily in terms of sexual attractiveness. As they become more aware of the role their bodies play in attracting the opposite[2] sex, the more attention they pay to specific features.

Other studies have looked into the gender differences and 'body satisfaction'. Offer *et al.* (1984) imply that social and cultural factors are of significance in how females express greater concern about their bodies. Maybe this is due to the fact that society still generally places greater importance on the female body. This is particularly obvious in the media, where women in advertisements are frequently depicted as thin 'body beautiful stereotypes'. The relationship between body-image and self-concept in late adolescence has shown that the female's self-esteem correlates with how attractive they find themselves, whereas males differentiate less about their attractiveness. The above findings suggest that for men, self-concept relate more to body attitudes and 'individual' physical effectiveness than to 'interpersonal' physical attractiveness.

Erikson (1968), by contrast placed major emphasis on the adolescent's physical attributes as a source of identity and self-concept. His theory is that the development of the personality and self-identity is dependent upon a fusion of individual biological, psychological and sociological components. In other words *"Each sex must view their bodies in a biologically appropriate, i.e. adaptive, manner so that complete synthesis and concomitantly successful self-definition can be achieved"*.

Sexuality, sex education and disability

Until recently, it was suggested that disabled adolescents were alienated, isolated and lonely and had little opportunity to share an emotional, physical or sexual relationship with either able-bodied or disabled people (Rieve 1989). Therefore, it was speculated that because of their isolation, disabled teenagers might lack opportunities to attend sex education classes and engage in social and sexual experimentation (Strax 1988).

In the western world, the number of children and adolescents surviving into adulthood with chronic, disabling conditions, has increased substantially over the last two decades (Blackburn 1995, Hallum 1995, Wolman and Basco 1994). Arguably, this may be due to technological advancements that have enabled children to survive prematurity, complex deliveries, foetal anomalies and other complicated diseases. Furthermore, as a result of improved clinical care, greater insight into the complexities of congenital anomaly, and easily accessible 'web site' international literature about chronic, childhood illnesses, many of the children who would have previously died in the 1970s, now survive into adolescence and

---

[2] I do not assume that all relationships are heterosexual.

Figure 3.4 Socialization and access to sex education

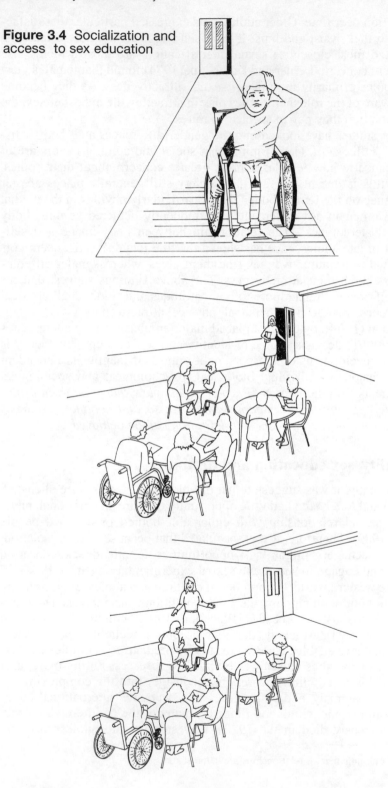

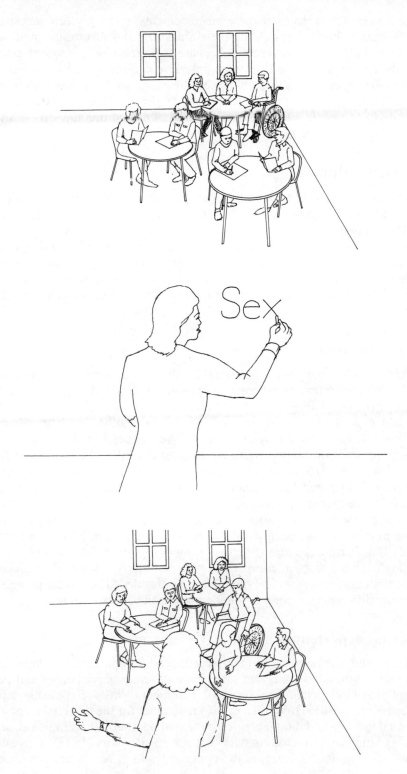

adulthood. Yet, in spite of these advancements, relatively few investigators have published results of their *Sexuality and Disability* inquiries. Why is this? Is it because researchers are concerned by society's response to their findings, or the dilemmas posed by publishing results in a cost-conscious society, without being able to guarantee definitive solutions? The limited number of publications may be perceived as a sad indictment on disabled people and may only serve to reinforce the unjustified myth that disabled people do not have sexual feelings.

Sexual attitudes

It is now recognized that health professionals should be adequately prepared if they are to advise or assist their clients with issues related to sexuality. In their study on knowledge and attitudes towards sexuality among pre-registration and registered nurses in New Zealand, Giddings and Wood (1998) found that nurses were often inadequately prepared to help clients with their concerns about sexual issues. These researchers compared their findings with other similar overseas studies undertaken in the 1990s.

Sex education

Until recently, many sex education classes were integrated with physical education programmes, where many physically disabled young people did not participate. Blum *et al.* (1991) noted that nearly half of all physically disabled adolescents did not receive sex education in their schools. Among those who did receive school sex education, less than 20% received any information pertinent to their disability. In one of the few published studies to include able-bodied 'controls' (like our own), Cromer *et al.* (1990) noted lower levels of sexual knowledge among teenagers with SB compared with non-disabled adolescents. Less than 20% of their 'spina bifida group' had sought advice about sexual or reproductive function in spite of expressing wishes to have children in adult life (see Figure 3.5). Furthermore, only 16% of Cromer's 'spina bifida' sample were using contraception, in comparison with 66% in the two control groups; one with cystic fibrosis and the other non-disabled. There were no age or gender differences among Cromer's sample and control groups.

Sexual experiences and activity

Haavik and Menninger (1981) observed that developmentally delayed and physically disabled teenagers often have different expectations and perceptions of independence and sexual fulfilment. Whilst relationship experiences may differ, Brookman (1986) noted that for the disabled teenager, sexual feelings and thoughts often increased. Dorner in his empirical, sexuality study of 63 teenagers with SB, age 13–19 years (1977), suggested that denying disabled people the opportunity to have sex did not necessarily suppress their sexual feelings. On the contrary, he noted that sexual interest was of a markedly preoccupying nature in young people with SB/HC. Such preoccupation's often increased with maturity and the total absence of a sexual partner could result in displays of 'inappropriate sexual behaviour', such as masturbating in public, or excessive requests for physical affection from a carer. Dorner also noted that although most of his sample had received some form of sex education, few had engaged in relationships or dated. Blum *et al.* 1991 have also concurred that the incidence of 'dating' among physically disabled adolescents is at variance with their able-bodied peers (Cromer *et al.* 1990). Generally the degree to which disabled adolescents engage in sexual activity remains unclear and sometimes produces conflicting results. Borjeson and Lagergren (1990) reported that adolescents with SB were less sexually active than their able-bodied peers. In contrast, Cromer *et al.* (1990) reported that about 25% of their disabled adolescents had had sexual experiences; including intercourse, and that the severity of their disability was not associated with sexual or social adjustment.

The Royal College of Nursing Sexuality Working Party published *Guidance for Nurses* about their duties and responsibilities in supporting disabled people with their sexual difficulties (RCN 2000). This group met following a Resolution debated at the RCN Congress in 1998 about the *Sexual rights of disabled people and the nurse's role*. The group included

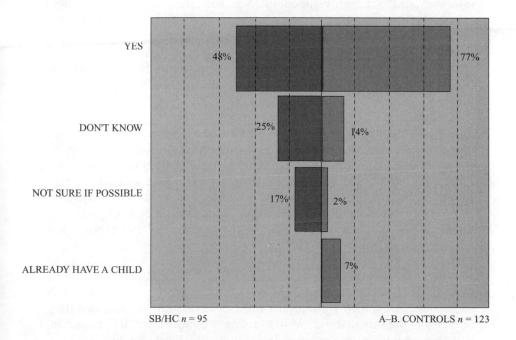

Figure 3.5 The desire to have children (from Cromer *et al.* 1990): the spina bifida/hydrocephalus group compared with a control group.

nurses who work in the spheres of learning disability, physical disability, sexual health, policy, law and disability. Since writing this text, the Department of Health have extended their work on sexuality.

Conclusion

In England and Wales it is recognized that sex education has a place in the curriculum for both disabled and able-bodied people. However, one of the greatest challenges is to decide *whose* individual responsibility it is to provide sex education. While many parents may be prepared to teach the basic facts of reproduction, many are reluctant to discuss other aspects of sexuality, such as intimate care procedures with their disabled adolescents. Equally, many teaching staff feel unhappy about providing specialist sex education for their students. All too often, the curriculum hinges on the more stereotypical aspects of sex education, such as pregnancy, contraception and childbirth. Little is focused on topics such as intimacy, touch, and alternative ways of receiving and giving sexual fulfilment, continence management during sexual activity and inappropriate sexual behaviours (Shapland 1999).

As society begins to acknowledge the rights of disabled people, some assurance that they will receive appropriate sex education, counselling and help when required, throughout adult life, must be given greater importance. The object of sex education should not be solely to provide information about bodily functions. Sex education should enable both able-bodied and disabled children to grow up feeling *"more confident about their sexuality and be able to make safer decisions about their lives and their relationships"* (Lenderyou 1993). Appropriate sex education should also be able to minimize some of the difficulties encountered by disabled people during adolescence and the transition period into adult life.

Encouraging disabled teenagers to establish their own sexual identity during adolescence is extremely important. At a time when socialization, independence, sexual awareness and experimentation increases in all young people, providing sex education and information about body image, self-esteem and socialization should be regarded as a normal part of adolescence, irrespective of whether one is able-bodied or 'disabled'.

All of us are sexual beings, whether or not we elect to express ourselves in this way. Sexuality – is about the way we feel and express ourselves, either as a man or woman, and how we relate to others physically, socially and emotionally. Individuals will have varying sexual needs and some will have stronger sexual feelings and desires than others. People with disabilities also have sexual feelings, although they may not always be able to express their feelings and in some cases may be prevented from doing so in the way that they would feel most comfortable. It is important that those advising or teaching disabled people about sex not only feel comfortable and are confident with the subject, but also have the ability to communicate effectively with the disabled person. People with SB generally have a normal sexual drive and sexual needs. It is therefore equally important that these young people learn about sex and sexual expression and can access good bladder and bowel advice, which are important for their socialization and sexual function from appropriately trained nursing and/or health care staff.

Research – methods and preliminary results

4

Background to the research

Dr Martin Bax and I were specifically invited by The Association of Spina Bifida and/or Hydrocephalus (ASBAH) to examine the sexual knowledge and experiences of young adults with spina bifida and/or hydrocephalus. This book primarily addresses the main findings of this research. In addition, some of the difficulties and dilemmas the research raised are discussed in Chapter 2, in the hope that they will provide assistance to other specialists who undertake sexual health work or research. The ethics of undertaking sexuality research proved as challenging and sensitive as obtaining the information about sexuality and disability itself.

ASBAH often receives inquiries for counselling and sex education from young disabled adults. As the need for sex education and the demand on ASBAH's disabled Living Advisory Service increased in the 1990s, they established a nation-wide sexual counselling service. This provided training courses for professionals, parents/carers as well as young people themselves. A former head of this service was keen to assess the benefits as well as review the Counselling service. I welcomed the challenge to undertake such research, knowing that these interviews were likely to be difficult and would require careful and sensitive management. Although I hoped that the information would generate fruitful results, I was also mindful that the research could lead to the disclosure of sensitive information. ASBAH felt that my previous training as a nurse and health visitor equipped me for this project. I requested and received additional specialist interview training prior to beginning the work.

Back in the 1980s, ASBAH in conjunction with SCOPE (formerly the Spastic Society) produced a sex education handbook. Although a unique, innovative and valuable publication for that time, ASBAH felt it required updating and revising to keep abreast with practice in the new millennium. The charity also felt that most people would prefer information in keeping with the latest technology; such as simple leaflets, videos, audiocassettes, diskettes, CD-ROMs and web pages.

Until the 1990s, information relating to sex education provision in schools and colleges as well as information about the physical and emotional needs of disabled people was generally limited. Much of the literature at the end of the last millennium examined sexual activity, function and dysfunction following traumatic or acquired injuries to the spinal cord. When a person has major bowel and/or urinary dysfunction combined with immobility, it is likely that this may affect sexual activity but not necessarily inhibit sexual desire. Naturally this may cause a disabled person to feel concerned, particularly in relation to his or her self-image and attractiveness to someone of the opposite or same sex. Being able to communicate as well as enjoy a physical or sexual relationship may be a major concern for the disabled person. Furthermore, physically disabled people sometimes feel alienated, isolated and lonely and may have infrequent opportunities to share an emotional, physical or sexual relationship, with either an able-bodied or disabled person. One aim of this work was to find out whether previous findings correlated with the experiences of this particular group of young disabled adults.

Although ASBAH agreed to fund the study, given the sensitivity of the subject matter, a feasibility study was first undertaken. An initial review of the international literature and some interviews were undertaken. The literature review is discussed in Chapter 3. In consultation with ASBAH's counselling service, the following aims and objectives for the study were agreed:

- To assess the disabled person's present knowledge and understanding of her or her own anatomy and physiology.
- To obtain information regarding any form of sex education that the young person had received either at school, college or elsewhere.
- To identify the sources of sex education, particularly if this had not been provided in a school or college.
- To identify individuals who may require initial or additional sex education.
- To find out the best ways of giving information about sex. Was it by formal teaching, leaflets, videos or one to one counselling?
- To assess how much the young person's disability impacted on his or her opportunity and ability to enjoy a 'sexual' relationship.
- To find out how many disabled people were having a relationship[1].
- To assess how many disabled people were engaged in a physical/sexual relationship with either a disabled or non-disabled person.
- To ascertain relationship preferences[2].

It was hoped that the feasibility study would offer some preliminary guidance for improving the delivery of sex education, if in fact it was found to be deficient.

---

[1] A physical relationship needs to be distinguished from a sexual one. This is discussed in Chapter 5.

[2] Physical and/or sexual relationship. Heterosexual, homosexual, bisexual. This is discussed in Chapter 6.

For the pilot study, twelve young adults, aged 16–25 years were randomly selected from three districts where I applied and had been granted local research ethics committee approval. The young people were matched for age, gender and social class. Six males and six females were invited to participate. Three females unfortunately declined on the grounds of shyness, embarrassment, and fear of ignorance and religion. However, one of the female's parents was particularly anxious for her daughter to participate. Only nine people ultimately participated in the pilot study.

The interview was divided into two sections, using a structured questionnaire schedule (see Appendix 2). Participants were invited to take part in both sections but could decline to continue after the first section, if they requested. Only one female declined to participate in the second part of the interview. Interviews were mainly conducted in the client's home or in residential centres. One person was interviewed in hospital. I considered asking both a specialist male interviewer and/or a specially trained disabled person to help with the interviews. However, the travelling and distance presented some practical difficulties, so at this stage, the former Head of ASBAH's counselling service (also female) and I carried out all the interviews. Reliability checks were made using Sex Education Training Cards, produced by the Family Planning Association.

Four males and five females were interviewed and one disabled couple elected to be interviewed together as they planned to marry in the near future. Eight out of nine of those interviewed were unemployed at the time, although two had previously worked: one man as a computer technician and one woman as a medical secretary. Two males and one female were training in a sheltered workshop and one male was a full-time university student. All the young people had spina bifida and hydrocephalus. In relation to religion, two people were Roman Catholics, one was a Muslim, one an Anglican and another a Salvationist. I felt it was important to ask the young person about their religion. A high refusal rate from particular religious groups might have influenced how we invited people to participate in any future studies. Furthermore, structuring the questions to suit different religions and cultures was considered an important feature of the questionnaire design.

Sexual knowledge and sex education

Part A of the interview included questions about sexual knowledge and sex education. Eight of the young adults said they had received sex education (see Table 4.1). Only three stated that their syllabus had included information about sexuality and disability. Five stated that their teaching had included the following subjects: conception, pregnancy and birth. Only three had received advice about contraception (see Table 4.2). Young adults who had attended The Chailey Heritage Residential School and John Groom's Residential Centre had received some sex education. Of note were the number of 'cannot remember' responses throughout the two-part interviews. This appeared indicative of some of the retentive memory difficulties that may be associated with hydrocephalus.

Table 4.1 Sources of sex education information received (total number of participants in sample: *n* = 9)

	Total
Parents	3
Relations	0
School/college lessons	7
Friends	4
Magazines/videos	3
Nurses	0
Social worker	3
GP	0
Hospital doctor	0
Day centre staff	1
Picked it up	4
Other	0
Don't know	0

Table 4.2 Sex education subjects requested (total number of participants: *n* = 9)

	Total
Puberty	5
Conception	5
Labour and confinement	5
Contraception	5
Basic child care	5
Infant feeding	6
Other subjects requested	
Sexuality	2
Sexual intercourse and disability	2
Emotional feelings during pregnancy	2

Three of the young people stated that they had a regular boy- or girl-friend. When asked if they would like to have children, two people reported that they were unsure. Three people were particularly concerned about the potential risks of disability to a baby, while two others were uncertain if they would be able to conceive or give birth. One young woman had already been pregnant and undergone a therapeutic abortion at 14 weeks. At the time of interview, she feared another pregnancy and accepted a referral by us to the hospital for advice. At this stage, she did not wish to use ASBAH's Psychosexual Counselling Service. Three people said they would consider pregnancy, subject to knowing more about the genetic risks. Seven of the sample felt that the risk of disability was a major deterrent to pregnancy[3].

Emotional experiences

The second part of the interview considered relationship experiences. The questionnaire schedule also asked questions about puberty. Throughout this section, Family Planning Association Sex Education Teaching Cards were used to facilitate information, maintain accuracy and reduce any embarrassment the young person might possibly feel about answering the questions. The young people were asked if they had heard of the following terms: 'puberty', 'menstruation', 'masturbation', 'erections' and 'wet dreams'. The majority stated that they had heard most of the terms except for 'wet dreams' and 'masturbation'. In two of the interviews, these particular questions were not asked because the individuals appeared to be shy. Defining terms provided a mixed response, many young people stating they could not define the terms (see Table 4.3). This raised our concerns about the possible impact of hydrocephalus on the young person's ability to recall information. One female said that she had received sex education teaching 3 weeks previously but was unable to recall much of the information she had been taught. One man said he had received regular sex education but that he frequently forgot the precise words, terms and their meanings. Four females knew that they had started their periods between 11–13 years. One young person 'did not know' as opposed to 'could not remember' when she had started to menstruate. Two females had monthly periods, one woman menstruated every second month, one less frequently and one did not know when her periods occurred, although she knew that she had periods! Most of the sample knew that periods occur at monthly intervals. The teaching cards largely elucidated appropriate responses for the anatomical body parts. 'Sperm', 'masturbation' and 'virgin' proved more difficult terms for the young people to define.

Two males stated that they had never had an erection, while two men had erections at other times of the day in addition to early morning erections. Another man said that he had infrequent early morning erections. Only two males experienced wet dreams. Two females had had full penetrative sexual intercourse. Seven of the sample stated that they would like to have sexual intercourse. Looking, touching, stroking, kissing, cuddling and petting were considered other natural ways of exciting one's partner. Three of the young adults declined to answer this particular question. All respondents interviewed felt they were heterosexual. One male had been

---

[3] Current figures record the incidence of spina bifida as 2 per 1000 live births, 1 in 35 infants being affected if one of the parents has spina bifida, and 1 in 10 if both parents have spina bifida (ASBAH Information Sheet 1 2001).

previously castrated because his penis had become gangrenous. He told us that he felt[4] confused about his personal sexual orientation and sexual preferences and was receiving counselling support.

Table 4.3 Young person's definition of terms (total number of participants: *n* = 9)

Sperm	A wriggly tadpole
	Liquid from penis
	Male gamete fertilizing female egg
	Do not know (2)
	Can't remember (2)
Virgin	Someone who has not kissed the opposite sex
	When a woman makes love to a man
	Having sex with someone
	Don't know (1)
	Can't remember (2)
Masturbation*	Making oneself happy
	Helping one's penis to become larger

*Seven subjects only asked.

Table 4.4 The following problems and anxieties related to intercourse were reported by the young people (total number of participants: *n* = 7)

Urinary incontinence	3
Urine bag leakage	2
Supra-pubic catheters	2
Faecal incontinence	2
Back pain and position	2
Fear of hurting partner, particularly through body weight	2
Finding a comfortable position	3
Sexual identity	1

So what did we learn from the early interviews?

It is difficult to draw firm conclusions with a sample size of only nine people. However, the young people did highlight some of the physiological aspects, sexual difficulties, limitations of sex education provision and

---

[4] *Felt*, as opposed to *stated*. In the larger study there were some ambiguous feelings discussed about sexual orientation.

relationship experiences for many disabled people (see Table 4.4). As most of the young people interviewed at this stage had hydrocephalus, it was felt that some consideration should be given for a larger study to explore the impact that hydrocephalus could have on learning, coding and retaining information about sex. On the basis of our report, ASBAH agreed that these initial results justified further investigation, and approved funding for a more detailed project with slight modifications. The revised aims were agreed as follows:

- To assess the disabled person's present knowledge and understanding of his/her own anatomy and physiology.
- To obtain information regarding any form of sex education that the young person had received either at school or college.
- To identify the source of sex education if this had not been provided in a school or college.
- To identify individuals who may require initial or additional sex education.
- To ascertain what was the best way to give information about sex? Was it by formal teaching, leaflets, videos or one to one counselling?
- To understand how much the young person's disability impacted on their opportunity and ability to enjoy a fulfilling, 'sexual' relationship.
- To establish how many disabled people were having a relationship[5].
- To establish how many disabled people were engaged in a physical/ sexual relationship with either a disabled or non-disabled person.
- To ascertain whether relationships[6] were preferred with disabled or non-disabled people.

In addition, it was hoped that I might make some assessment on the impact of hydrocephalus on the young person's ability 'to store' and recall information about sexual information[7]. Mindful that young people did not want the results only presented in report form, ASBAH were keen that there should be some practical outcomes from this work such as:

- Recommendations for improving the delivery of sex education if found deficient.
- Offering advice on methods of enjoying a fulfilling relationship within the boundaries of the young person's disability, age, religious beliefs and preferred relationships (personal sexual orientation).
- Design and production in conjunction with young disabled people, suitable education materials based on the key findings from the study.

Such interviews naturally generated feelings in the young people we had interviewed. I was conscious that a careful and skilled explanation of the

---

[5] Physical relationship needs to be separated from a sexual one. This is discussed in Chapter 5.

[6] Physical and/or sexual relationship.

[7] At this stage I engaged the services of a clinical psychologist, part-time, to assist us with this task.

study was required before interview and this was offered. Furthermore, I left time at the end of both sections of interview to allow for further discussion and clarification of any particular points. I always provided the contact number of a Counselling Service for future reference or counselling support. Where interviews were conducted in a hospital ward, a follow-up visit was offered by a trained counsellor to ensure that the young person had not felt embarrassed by the interview and had the opportunity to reflect and seek further information, if requested. Only two people requested follow-up visits. This was mainly to obtain further information about sexuality and disability.

The main research project

Oliver (1990, 1992) and Zarb (1992) questioned the appropriateness of 'Disability' research being undertaken by able-bodied people. In 1990, Professor Michael Oliver argued that disabled people see research as irrelevant, failing to respond and improve their overall quality of life and circumstances, if undertaken by people who may not understand particular issues facing disabled people. Mindful of these comments, this study's advisory panel included both able-bodied and disabled people (see Acknowledgements and Chapter 1). Advisory panel members were invited to discuss the ethical and practical issues of the project, advise on its development and monitor the able-bodied researchers' ability to handle interviews and analysis about sensitive and delicate matters.

Action research

The object of most social research is to investigate a particular or series of questions, make possible recommendations and prove or refute the original hypothesis/hypotheses. The researcher is not usually responsible for initiating policy change but the outcome of such research may lead to policy reforms.

The person undertaking 'action' or 'evaluative research' hopes to *"monitor and possibly to evaluate its effect both before and after change has taken place and not just test hypotheses"* McNeill (1992).

My decision to undertake 'action research' stems from the research philosophies described by Barnes (1992), Oliver (1992) and Professor of Nursing, Christine Webb (1989). In this respect, the researcher hopes to contribute to the empowerment of disabled people through partnership and reciprocity. It is inherent to action research philosophy that study objectives are of mutual benefit to both participants and the researcher. If these objectives are mutually acceptable, researchers may benefit from developing skills and knowledge while participants may be empowered to influence some fundamental changes concerning their own lives. The following statement made during one of the early 'pilot' interviews strengthens the argument for reciprocity.

If this is yet another report, full of jargon and left to gather dust on an inaccessible shelf, then I'm not interested! If the research will produce practical materials and solutions as a priority ... then the survey (study) will have served its purpose! (woman with spina bifida)

Similar comments were voiced by other disabled adults.

Action research has recently enjoyed increasing popularity across various disciplines, but particularly among nurse researchers (Holter and Schwartz-Barcott 1993, Webb 1989). Webb suggests that this results from limitations within both quantitative and qualitative research methods. She argues that both approaches may disservice the participant. This is apparent in research where sensitive issues, such as sex, may be discussed but the problems identified are often ignored.

The relationship may be seen to be one-sided, hierarchical, with the 'respondent' giving generously of his or her time and the researcher using the data but being unable to reciprocate (see Chapter 2). If nursing research is about caring and partnership, then collaborative discussion within the boundaries of the client's cognitive capabilities must be considered.

Action Research has also been deployed in education and community development programmes since the 1960s (McNeill 1992). For example, the Plowden Report (HMSO 1967) examined the state of Britain's primary schools and noted that education standards were considerably lower in certain urban areas. This led to the formation of Educational Party Areas (EPAs) where additional funding was allocated to primary schools in disadvantaged areas, hoping to empower and offer these children the same educational opportunities as their peers living in more privileged communities.

Ethnographic research: is this better for disabled people?

Ethnography or qualitative research describes *"the culture and life style of the group of people being studied, in a way that is as faithful as possible to the way they see it themselves"* (McNeill 1992). This form of research enquiry is concerned with 'individual meaning and interpretation'. It is distinct from quantitative methodology, which is more concerned with statistical objectivity (Barnes 1992). Statistical logic and experimentation do not necessarily provide opinions or definitive answers from 'objective experts' or help people to learn about society (Barnes 1992).

The ethnographic approach is frequently used in smallscale studies, or in complex, sensitive, emotional research (Moser and Kalton 1979) such as this. The researcher has personal contact with the social world, particularly its 'social life within its natural context' (Barnes 1992). This method offers both the interviewer and interviewee greater flexibility during the research interview, particularly in addressing individual questions (Barnes 1992). The interviewee is encouraged to dictate the pace, development and content of the interview(s), and the researcher is obliged to reconsider issues which he or she may have overlooked within the original research strategy. Ethnographic interviews often succeed in eliciting information, particularly of a sensitive nature, where other methods may fail. It is frequently selected for people with learning difficulties or for those who may find difficulty completing and/or answering structured questionnaires. Sometimes referred to as the 'non-directive, in depth or non-guided interview' (Clark and Robinson 1989), the informant is encouraged to talk about him or herself in the context of the subject matter, in this case sex. A semi-structured interview schedule questionnaire may be used to facilitate discussion.

Quantitative research

Quantitative research is more accustomed to emphasizing the importance of statistics and objectivity (see Barnes 1992, Stanley 1991) than examining the individual, personal circumstances of a group or groups of people.

Survey data is usually collected either through postal questionnaires or structured, 'face to face' interviews (Rogers 1988).

The advantages of postal questionnaires are:

1. Cost effectiveness
2. Privacy and personal convenience
3. Probability of collecting larger samples over a wider geographical area (if this is a specific aim of the study)
4. Anonymity
5. Time to consider the questions
6. Autonomy.

Postal questionnaires may be difficult for disabled people to complete for the following reasons:

1. Recipients may require assistance to complete them
2. The intended recipient may not receive the questionnaire
3. Correspondence may be opened by someone else, sometimes without the intended recipient's knowledge
4. Sensitive research may be more suitably discussed in a direct interview
5. Postal questionnaires often evoke a poor response among elderly and disabled people.

Interviews addressing the subject of sexuality and disability conducted with disabled people are usually better when they are face-to-face, to allow opportunities for discussion and clarification, if necessary. I also hoped that it would establish greater trust and confidence in the research if the disabled person met me.

A well-designed questionnaire is written so that the respondent will immediately understand what is required. Adults with cognitive deficits may need reminding and offered guidance about answering some questions. A structured questionnaire may help the researcher to focus the inquiry. This is especially important for adults with poor concentration or who exhibit 'cocktail party syndrome' behaviour, which was a feature of some of the people who took part in this study.

Observational diaries: A third alternative?

Robert E. Park, an American Sociologist (1864–1944), developed 'participant observation' during his studies of the deviant behaviour of 'hoboes' (tramps) and gang-members living in Chicago. In this method, the researcher observes the social processes of a group or groups of individuals, makes personal notes and uses case histories in order to create a total picture of the research question(s) (McNeill 1992). In Britain, Madge and Harrison (1939) in their 'Mass Observation' studies, used both participant and non-participant observation, diaries, reports and case histories. The object of their research was based on 'observation of everyone, by everyone including themselves' and culminated in an extraordinary project addressing the everyday lives of ordinary people. Although observational diaries were not the main methods used in this study, they were used to support the ethnographic approach. 'Observation' may assist the researcher working with learning disabled people, who may have communication difficulties. This method may also help to corroborate information collected by questionnaire and/or interview and ultimately assist in validating survey data.

The study which adopts a varied methodology may display different features and qualities and overcome the individual limitations of any one method. Quantitative surveys may display reliability and representativeness while omitting crucial points because a questionnaire can only answer what is asked. Ethnography provides validity and sensitivity but may lack reliability (McNeill 1992). Diaries and observation 'provide a richness of detail' but may result in some research bias (Moser and Kalton 1979).

Whilst the selection of an appropriate methodology may be intrinsic to research development and outcome, the principles of reciprocity and empowerment of disabled people (Zarb 1992) cannot be ignored, particularly in research about the sexuality of disabled people.

Background to this study

As previously stated, The Association for Spina Bifida and Hydrocephalus (ASBAH) receives numerous requests for counselling support and sex education from young disabled adults. In conjunction with the former Spastics Society (SCOPE), ASBAH produced a sex education handbook which was revised in 1983. Leaflets and videos are now generally preferred.

In 1990, ASBAH established a nationwide counselling service for young adults, their families and carers, in response to an increasing number of requests for sex education information and sexual counselling.

In addition, they wanted to know what were the difficulties about sex education? Were they due to lack of, or inappropriate, sex education, or the possible effect of hydrocephalus on recalling the information? Was the ASBAH counselling service efficacious?

ASBAH hoped that the information would provide suitable guidelines for service development and identify educational needs for these clients, their carers, and professionals.

Ethical committee approval

Approval for these studies was ultimately granted from all local Research Ethics Committees within 5 months of application (total=23 research ethics committees). The ethical considerations of this study have previously been discussed in Chapter 2.

Pilot study

To assess the feasibility of this study, a random sample of twelve young adults, aged 16–25 years (mean age 23.5 years) with spina bifida and/or hydrocephalus, were invited to participate. They were selected from three of the twenty-three districts (Kent=6, North West Thames Region=17) where ethics committees had approved the research proposal.

The pilot study provided illustrative, as opposed to definitive, data but was sufficiently important to precipitate the development of a larger and more comprehensive study.

Identifying the sample

A sample of all the people with SB/HC known to the following organizations was selected for this study from the following sources:

1. ASBAH's counselling and fieldwork service.
2. Former Westminster (Children's) Hospital Medical Records Department.
3. Family Fund (Social Policy Research Unit, York University).

The sample was randomly selected from all the people on the above-listed databases. Adults with spina bifida, both with or without hydrocephalus were included but adults with only hydrocephalus were excluded. The focus of this research was on adults with spina bifida with hydrocephalus, rather than hydrocephalus alone. It was felt that the aforementioned sampling frames were more likely to be accurate and complete as these organizations provided services and were in regular contact with this population. Because of the sensitive subject matter, we were particularly concerned to avoid inappropriate contact with young adults, particularly those with severe learning difficulties or who were very unwell.

The sample

Kent (K) districts and the North West Thames Region (NWTR) were selected because of their proximity to London, health services provided in these districts[8] and ASBAH's specific requests for these locations. Sixty-two young adults from Kent and an equivalent number of young adults with SB/HC from NWTR were invited to participate. The samples were matched for age, gender and (parental) social class (see Table 4.5).

Table 4.5 Parents' occupation–social class compared with local population

OPCS classification		SB/HC (%)	Able-bodied (%)
I.	Professional	2	11
II.	Intermediate	13	13
III.	Non-manual	25	12
III.	Manual	36	11
IV.	Semi-skilled	11	5
V.	Unskilled	5	0
	Housewife	4	1
Non-respondents		4	48

SB/HC, spina bifida/hydrocephalus; OPCS, Office of Population Censuses and Surveys (Now known as the Office for National Statistics, London).

There were particular reasons for including Kent within the sample. Specific concerns had been raised about the lack of sexual knowledge of people with SB living in this county. ASBAH was keen to see if Kent's views were representative of other districts. Time, manpower and limited finances prevented other districts in the South East from being included. All districts within the North West Thames region were included.

Reliability of sample source

Incidence rates for spina bifida have fallen considerably since the 1960s (when the majority of this SB/HC population resident in the UK were born). There are innumerable geographical and temporal variations of SB/HC throughout the United Kingdom.

Few cases of SB have recently been notified for residents living in and around London (ASBAH 2001). This would suggest a low rate of people with spina bifida and hydrocephalus in this area. Different data sources

---

[8] Specialist clinics at the former Westminster Children's Hospital, now part of the Chelsea and Westminster Hospital, Imperial College London.

yield variable sample sizes. The ASBAH and hospital databases appeared to be more reliable than those of the Family Fund.

Making comparisons?

I intended to compare the SB/HC sample data with young adults who had another disability, for example cerebral palsy (CP). Adults with cerebral palsy share many of the physiological and neurological features as people with SB/HC. People with CP had expressed similar concerns about their sexuality and disability as those with spina bifida (SCOPE). Ten young adults with CP, of similar age and from the same regions were interviewed, but due to a poor response rate, this information is not discussed here.

Able-bodied people

The sexuality of able-bodied adults also begs discussion and further research. Sex education has heightened awareness but not necessarily changed the behaviour of able-bodied adolescents. One hundred and twenty-three able-bodied students age 16–25 years from two co-educational colleges of further education and three sixth forms within the two regions (School 1 $n=6$, School 2 $n=12$, School 3 $n=15$; co-educational: College 1 $n=50$, college 2 $n=40$) were interviewed to provide some normative control comparison with the spina bifida population. The controls were matched, in as far as this was possible, for age, geographical location, registrar general's social class classification and educational ability. However, the control data is not detailed within this text.

Comments on the disabled sample methods

The study took 3 months for over 50% of the local research ethics committees to give their approval. One committee reached its decision after 5 months. This resulted in some delay in initiating the study.

All adults over the age of 18 were asked to give written consent (Ethics Committee recommendations). All adults within the sample and control group were sent an explanatory letter, outlining the aims and objectives of the study, and offering preliminary interviews, information or telephone calls to provide further clarification about the study.

Six of the SB/HC sample requested preliminary interviews; two requested parental presence, while three parents asked to be present at interview(s) before allowing their son or daughter to take part. Six parents of the SB/HC group opened their son or daughter's mail and refused consent on their behalf, without showing the correspondence to their son or daughter. Two females, living in residential care, who initially declined to take part, later changed their minds, having observed me with other people in the centre. Ninety-eight of the SB/HC group and 123 of the control group agreed to participate in the structured interview (see Figure 4.1). One hundred adults with SB/HC were interviewed but two of the sample were subsequently excluded from the final analysis, as one person had primary hydrocephalus and another did not fit the age criteria, i.e. was over 25 years of age.

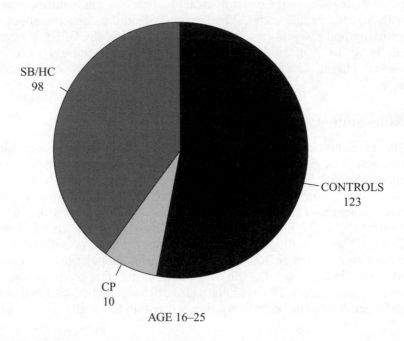

SB/HC
98

CONTROLS
123

CP
10

AGE 16–25

Figure 4.1 Numbers of study participants. CP, cerebral palsy; SB/HC, spina bifida/hydrocephalus

Response rate

The overall response rate from those with SB was 68%. Female responses in both the sample and control groups was higher (see Figure 4.2). Disabled people gave the following reasons for not taking part in the study: 'embarrassment', 'this does not apply to me', 'I know it all already', 'fear of ignorance', 'shyness'.

The control group: methods and problems

Several schools and colleges within the defined study area were contacted, with poor response rates. All heads of the schools and colleges and their governing bodies were sent letters outlining the aims and objectives of the study. Preliminary talks were given to staff and prospective par-

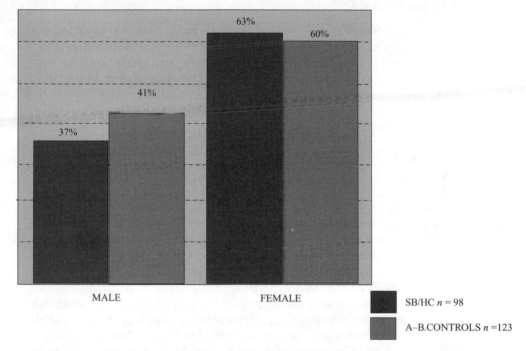

Figure 4.2 Response rate by gender. A.-B. = able-bodied

ticipants in all schools and colleges in advance of interviews. Obtaining permission to interview able-bodied controls proved problematic. There were particular difficulties in recruiting able-bodied males. Forty per cent (able-bodied males) and 60% (able-bodied females) took part (*n*=123: total controls, all districts). The schools and colleges included:

- **School 1** – fifty boys were invited. Twenty initially consented but only six agreed to be interviewed.
- **School 2** – twenty young men and women were invited. Four men and eight women consented.
- **School 3** – thirty (equal numbers of males and females) were invited. Ten men and five young women were interviewed.
- **College 1** – fifty young men and fifty women were invited. The response rate was high in females (44) but poor in males (6).
- **College 2** – twenty-five men and twenty-five women were invited. Eighteen men and twenty-two women responded.

Reasons for refusal included: "Shyness about a personal interview", "I know it already", "it's my business", "fear of disclosure of information to parents and staff".

The interviews

I was the principal interviewer. Reliability interviews were carried out on six people with SB. The ASBAH counselling coordinator interviewed two of the people with SB. A male university student with SB/HC was also given interview training. Travel, access and ultimately some personal difficulties prevented him from interviewing people. He advised on questionnaire design and development of some of the training materials.

The structured questionnaire

The questionnaire design was adapted from earlier research designed by Thomas *et al.* (1989) with ASBAH's assistance. It was divided into two sections (see Appendix 2) and designed to be self-administered or completed by the researcher during interview. Generally, the disabled people preferred someone to help them complete the questionnaires, as this allowed more opportunity to focus on the questions being asked, rather than having to concentrate on their writing skills (many people with spina bifida and/or hydrocephalus experience difficulty with handwriting). All adults were encouraged to answer both sections of the interview schedule, but were advised that completing one or other section was equally acceptable. Part A of the questionnaire addressed sex education, terminology and location of information (for example: school, college, peers, published literature, e.g. leaflets, etc.) Part B addressed personal relationship experiences, family planning, within its broadest context, genetic counselling and continence concerns (see Appendix 2).

The in-depth interview

Twenty out of the 100 adults with SB/HC and twenty able-bodied people were randomly selected from Kent and the North West Thames Region to take part in a semi-structured interview. Sixteen people with SB/HC and fifteen able-bodied people agreed to take part in this interview. They were, in so far as it was possible, matched for gender, social class and geographical compatibility. These interviews aimed to elicit sensitive information that the structured questionnaire might overlook. Five males and eleven females with SB/HC, and five able-bodied males and ten able-bodied females took part. All interviews were carried out by myself. The interviews never exceeded an hour. Mean average length of interview was 25 minutes. Interviews were transcribed 'word for word' by a part-time research assistant and myself. Transcripts included non-words (e.g. 'um's' and 'er's' and pauses). The accuracy of the written transcript was checked against the tape. All interviewees were offered a copy of the tape or transcript.

Both the sample and control groups were asked to discuss the following four questions:

1. What does Friendship mean to you?
2. What does Love mean to you?

3. What does a Relationship mean to you?
4. What does Sex mean to you?

Many of the sample group volunteered additional information to the four questions. The control group only agreed to answer the four specified questions. The definitions are outlined in Appendix 5.

Tools

These included a portable tape recorder and a supply of blank audio tapes to be used during ethnographic interviews. A notebook and pencil for diary observation were also available. Two sets of male/female anatomy cards, produced by the Family Planning Association, were used in both the structured and ethnographic interviews. The cards were particularly helpful for young people who were shy about answering certain questions and preferred to point to the answers on the card. One set of cards comprised several A4 illustrations of the male and female anatomy (such as Figure 4.3). A second set of cards was designed in the form of a jigsaw puzzle. This design enabled the young person to attach the appropriate piece of the jigsaw to the puzzle.

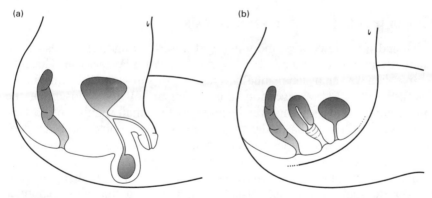

Figure 4.3 Samples from the set of cards used in the interview

Cognitive assessments

Assessing the cognition and ability to learn and code new information was thought to be of fundamental importance in this study, particularly for those adults who had HC as well as SB. Literature addressing the cognitive function of people with SB/HC has largely concentrated on the global assessment of intellectual ability (Cull and Wyke 1984). These authors noted that children with spina bifida and or hydrocephalus when compared with those of 'normal intelligence' showed deficits in their 'ability to learn, store and retrieve information'. The young person's hospital medical records in this study provided limited information about the young person's cognitive assessment or educational attainment. The structured interviews ultimately elicited the latter information. A clinical psychologist administered psychology tests on a random sample of eight adults with SB/HC.

Psychology assessment tools

The three assessment tools used were:

1. Wechsler Adult Intelligence Scale Revised (WAIS-R) (Wechsler, 1984).
2. Neale Analysis of Reading Ability (Neale, 1989).
3. Wechsler Memory Scales (WMS-R) (Wechsler, 1987).

These tests aimed to obtain the following information from the adults with SB/HC:

- An indication of their knowledge.
- Some comparison of their performance with individuals of the same age.
- To identify their strengths and weaknesses.
- To test verbal versus performance differences.
- Assess accuracy and comprehension of reading and the ability to learn using new verbal materials.

Ethnographic interviews: analysis

All taped interviews were individually transcribed and responses coded manually into a computer and indexed into a Word Perfect file. The subjective data was analysed manually. The data was thought to be unsuitable for SPSS PC PLUS conversion (the statistical software chosen for the Quantitative analysis). This was because of the small number of participants within this section of the study. Individual responses were categorized and grouped in order to discard irrelevancies and summarize the information and attempt to draw some conclusions.

The information was analysed using frequency distributions. Univariate analysis was only used to elicit information about singular variables. Some of the data was classified into non-numerical categories, such as marital status and occupation. The remainder were grouped into numerical categories.

Coding and statistics: quantitative study

The majority of questions were 'closed-ended' (where the answers have a fixed range of permitted responses, e.g. 'yes' or 'no'). This format may facilitate statistical analysis (Frude 1987). 'Closed' responses were translated into a coding format which is ideal for use with the statistical software SPSS PC PLUS. This statistical package was used for this section of the study. A research fellow with statistical expertise advised me.

A coding frame for the questionnaire was devised so that 'yes' or 'no' or the permitted responses were allocated numerical values. These were usually numbers between 1 to 8 (0 or 9 corresponding to 'not answered' or 'missing data'). Open-ended questions were kept to a minimum as they are difficult to analyse (Frude 1987). Suitable numerical values were ascribed to the few open-questions asked in Part B of the questionnaire. After coding, the raw data was entered into the computer in matrix form and given suitable variable names and labels.

Statistical analysis

The data for this study was classified mainly into a nominal scale (data is grouped into name classes), where categories are usually allocated a numerical coding and there is no formal mathematical relationship (Frude 1987). For this reason, most of the data was analysed through the computation of frequencies and cross-tabulations only. Number frequencies were allocated to the value of each specified variable in addition to the percentage totals. Cross-tabulations or contingencies show the distribution of frequencies of cases on more than two discrete variables (Frude 1987).

The Chi-squared test, which is used in non-parametric statistics, seemed appropriate to use for the analysis of some of this study's nominal data (the Chi-square is a statistical test which indicates whether the observed pattern of results would differ significantly, had they only occurred by chance). Unless otherwise stated, the level of statistical significance used was $P<0.01$.

5 What did we learn?

For ease of reference, findings are divided into three sections and their implications addressed separately. The results include quantitative, qualitative feedback and information from a small sample of young people who agreed to undertake some psychology tests.

Findings from the structured interview

This section focuses on the specific concerns of adults with spina bifida and/or hydrocephalus (SB/HC) but makes some comparison with the information obtained from able-bodied people, from now on referred to as the able-bodied control group (ABC group). Much of the information is cross-referenced with tables. The structured sexuality questionnaire is in Appendix 2 and the two sexuality coding frames are located in Appendix 3. The structured interview results are presented in two sections.

Part A of the structured questionnaire compared the 'sexual knowledge' of both the disabled group, from now on referred to as SB/HC and the control group (ABC). *Part B* compared 'relationship experiences' and puberty of both the able-bodied and disabled groups. Discussion only focuses here on the 'knowledge' and 'experiences' of adults with SB/HC.

The overall response rate was 68% (SB/HC) compared with 49% (ABC). Female responses were significantly higher in both the sample (63%) and control groups (60%) (see Figure 4.2 in the previous chapter). Ninety-one per cent of those with SB/HC had hydrocephalus. Fifty-five per cent of young adults with SB/HC were interviewed at home, the remainder in residential settings or other locations requested by the young people. All of the control group were interviewed in colleges or schools.

Part A of the structured questionnaire

Sexual knowledge results

Eighty per cent of young people with SB/HC compared with 94% of the ABC group stated that they had received sex education at school. Only 18% of young people with both SB/HC compared with 7% of young people with HC had received specific information about sexuality and

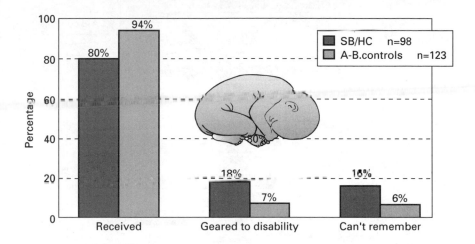

Figure 5.1 Nature of sex education received

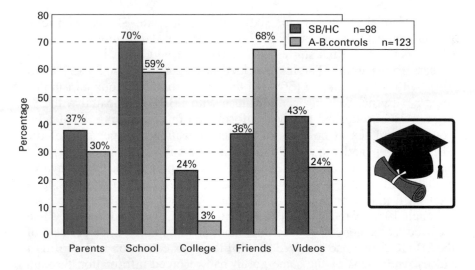

Figure 5.2 The main sources of sex education received

disability. Sixteen per cent of those with SB/HC compared with 6% of the young able-bodied people could not recall receiving any sex education (see Figure 5.1).

Sources of sex education

Figures 5.2 and 5.3 set out the main sources of sex education received from parents, school, college, peers, audio-visual and other sources from both the sample and control groups. School provided most information for both the sample and controls; 70% of the SB/HC group compared

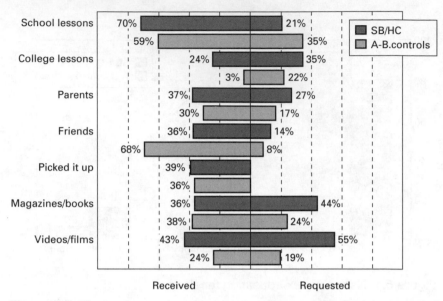

Figure 5.3 The main sources of sex education: received and requested

with 59% of the ABC group. Sixty-three adults with SB/HC who took part in Stephen Dorner's study (1977) reported similar results; twenty-one of the teenagers in his study had received sex education in school and fifteen from parents. Parents provided sex education for 36 (37%) of those with SB/HC and 37 (30%) of the ABC group who took part in this research. Twenty-four per cent of those with SB/HC compared with 3% of the ABC group had received information or counselling about relationships and sex at colleges of further education. Six per cent of the SB/HC group had requested information about sex, relationships and marriage from a sexual counsellor. Those with spina bifida and/or hydrocephalus had received little or no sex education from other relatives, hospital staff, family doctors, care staff, or social workers (see Figure 5.4), although 19% of the young people with SB/HC reported that they had received 'some genetic counselling' from doctors. Forty-three per cent of the SB/HC group had received most of their sex education in the form of videos while 36% of the same group had received information through books: this also included leaflets and magazines (see Figures 5.2 and 5.3).

Preferred information sources
Fifty-five per cent of young people with SB/HC would prefer to receive sex education in the form of videos compared with 19% of the ABC group (see Figure 5.3). The SB/HC group gave the following reasons for their preference of video materials:

* Dislike and difficulty in reading the written word.
* Able to look at video material more than once in order to reinforce their own learning.

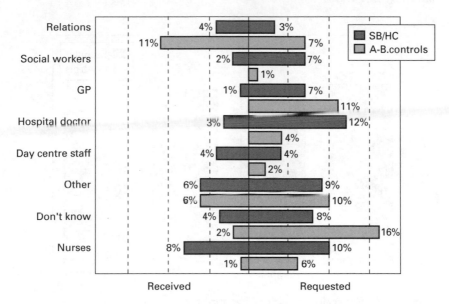

Figure 5.4 Sex education received versus sources/subjects requested

- Able to select video or particular sections of materials appropriate to their individual needs.
- Convenience. Able to view materials in privacy, either with or without a partner/friend and/or carer. (This was particularly important for those adults who were living independently or continued to be supported by parents/carers either at home or in residential care after leaving school.)
- Less embarrassing than discussing a topic among a large group of people.
- Wider choice of materials, including both sex education and certificate 18 or 'blue movies'. Thirteen of the sample said they regularly watched 'certificate 18' movies in order to obtain information, but also to relieve sexual frustration and boredom in the absence of a regular partner.

Simple leaflets and magazines were generally preferred by 44% of the disabled group. The young adults generally preferred information that had visual images and less text.

Information requested
Although both the disabled young people and the ABC groups had received information about conception, the length of pregnancy, birth/labour and birth control (see Figures 5.5 and 5.6), the SB/HC group requested further information about labour (54%), contraception (50%) and conception (46%). The sample group were particularly concerned to know whether their disability would affect potency (particularly the males), if the women could become pregnant, have a 'normal birth' or

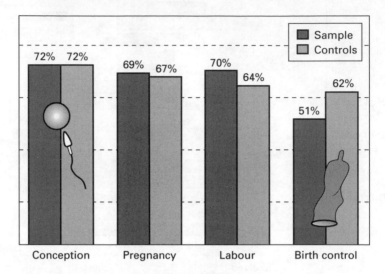

Figure 5.5 Sex education topics taught

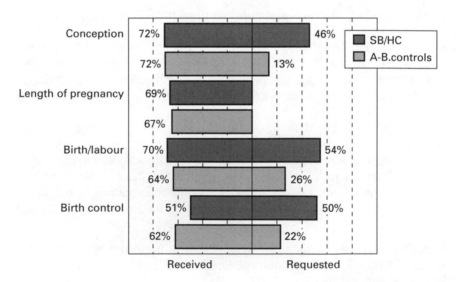

Figure 5.6 Sex education received versus sources/subjects requested

would require an instrumental birth, for example, a caesarean section. Both men and women in the sample group inquired about the use of contraceptive pills and condoms. Four men who used penile urinal sheaths wondered whether, in addition they also needed to use a condom. Figure 5.6 illustrates some of the specific information requests from the SB/HC sample. There were additional, individual requests and concerns, arising from one of the open ended questions about continence (*n*=13), sexual intercourse (*n*=13), society's attitude towards the sexuality of disabled people (*n*=9).

Knowledge of terms

Both groups had heard of and could explain the following anatomical terms and their functions: 'breasts', 'nipples' and 'penis' (Table 5.1). There were notable differences, however, among the disabled young people, between those who had heard, could offer definitions and understand some of these terms. Table 5.1 and Figures 5.7–5.10 illustrate some of the differences among the young people who had heard, could define and understand the different anatomical terms. Seventy-six per cent of those with SB/HC had heard the word 'vagina', only 69% of the group knew the correct definition, and 66% understood what it meant. Two

Table 5.1 Knowledge of terms

	Group	Heard (%)	Define (%)	Rate (%)
Puberty	SB/HC	78	65	57
	ABC	98	98	60
Period/ menstruation	SB/HC	86	46	
	ABC	95	49	
Virgin	SB/HC	63	52	50
	ABC	98	98	63
Vagina	SB/HC	76	69	66
	ABC	98	97	63
Function of nipples	SB/HC	74		70
	ABC	97		63
Where penis	SB/HC	81	78	75
	ABC	96	97	63

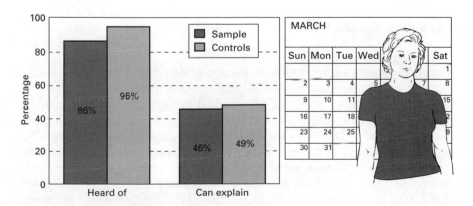

Figure 5.7 Knowledge of terms: 'period'

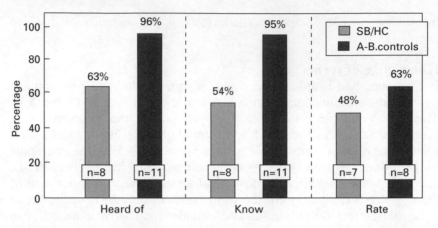

Figure 5.8 Knowledge of terms: 'erection'

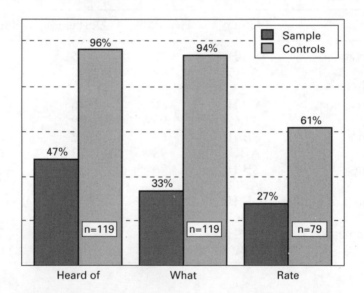

Figure 5.9 Knowledge of terms: 'wet dreams'

people thought a vagina was a 'non-meat eater'! The difference between hearing and understanding terms was evident in most of the SB/HC results. However, some of the able-bodied group expressed some difficulty in rating terms. Ninety-six per cent of the ABC group had heard the term penis, but only 63% of the ABC group understood the meaning. The author appreciates that some of the questions may have caused embarrassment, and resulted in some hesitant replies. Defining 'masturbation', 'erections' and 'wet dreams' proved particularly difficult (see Figures 5.8–5.10). Sixty-three per cent of the SB/HC group had heard the word 'erection' but only 48% understood what it meant. Eight of the SB/HC

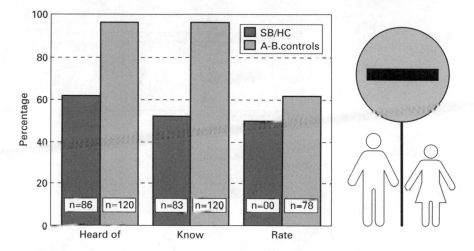

Figure 5.10 Knowledge of terms: 'virgin'

group thought 'wet dreams' were associated with urinary incontinence rather than ejaculation of sperm. Six of the SB/HC group who understood the terms 'erection' and 'masturbation' asked if it was 'wrong' or 'sinful' to 'masturbate'. Six male SB/HC adults requested advice about 'masturbation' and 'having erections'. Although 24% of the male sample 'thought' they had erections, only 21% said that their erections occurred more than once a day. Three men with SB/HC stated that they used to have early morning erections but these had ceased after they were 16 years of age.

Part B of the structured sexuality questionnaire

Puberty
Seventy-eight per cent of the SB/HC group compared with 98% of the ABC had heard the term puberty but only 57% of those with SB/HC, compared with 60% of the ABC group, understood the meaning of puberty. Fifteen per cent of those with SB/HC stated that their own puberty had started between 7–10 years of age, compared with 13% of the ABC group (see Figure 5.11). Forty-four per cent of the SB/HC group compared with 71% of the ABC group, began puberty between 11 and 13 years. Only 3% of the SB/HC group started puberty after 16 years. The able-bodied young people had all started puberty before 16 years. Fifteen per cent of women with SB/HC compared with 5% of ABC group had their menarche between 7–10 years (Figure 5.12). Members of the SB/HC group reported irregularities in the frequency of their periods, only 29% having monthly periods compared with 53% of able-bodied controls (see Figure 5.13).

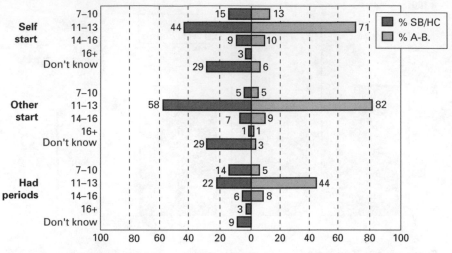

Figure 5.11 Puberty: knowledge and experiences

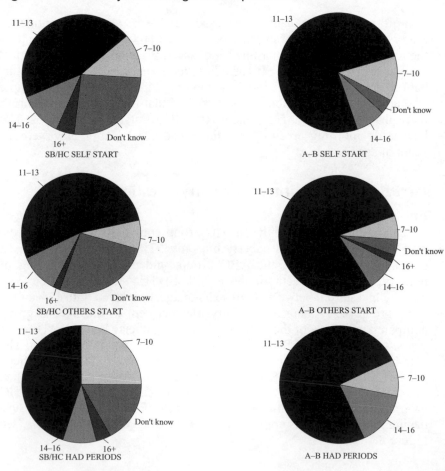

Figure 5.12 Puberty: knowledge and experiences

Relationships

Thirty-nine per cent of the SB/HC group compared with 55% of the ABC group reported that they previously had or were presently in a relationship, 'steady or long-term'. The definition of 'steady or long term relationship' used in this research was a relationship that had lasted for three months or longer (see Figure 5.14). Considerably more of the sample, 41% compared with only 16% of the ABC expressed concerns about 'long-term relationships'. There was some initial confusion as to what constituted a 'relationship'and it was clear that I needed to seek young people's views on this. Four women reported 'crushes' on teachers or taxi drivers and inappropriately interpreted the 'crush' as a physical or emotional relationship of long duration, particularly if the infatuation had lasted for more than a couple of years. Two men and one woman living in residential care were so obsessed by their care assistants/teachers that either the disabled person or their care assistant was reallocated other clients, moved to another area of the building or moved premises. Three of the disabled group reported that they had had homosexual relationships (two of the homosexual men took part in the qualitative interviews). A third homosexual male advised me that he was HIV positive and receiving treatment.

Forty-eight per cent of the SB/HC group compared with 77% of the ABC group wanted to have a child. Forty-two per cent of the SB/HC group were either ambivalent or uncertain about having a child. Although only 21% of the SB/HC group compared with 68% of the ABC group stated that they had had penetrative sex, 48% of the SB/HC group, compared with 71% of the ABC group would like to have the opportunity to make love. This question raised many issues about love-making, such as comfortable positions, etc. (see Figure 5.15). Penetrative sex was

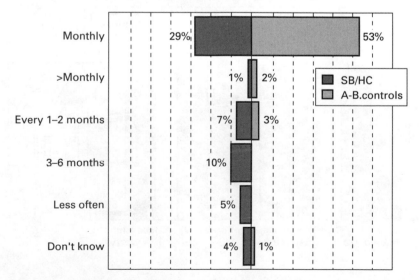

Figure 5.13 Menstrual period frequency

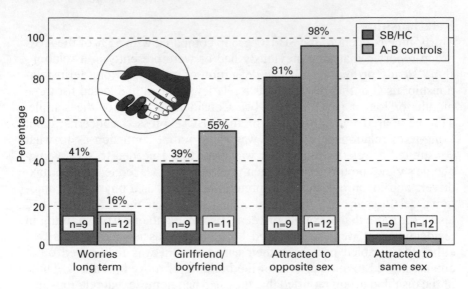

Figure 5.14 Steady or long-term relationships

not considered to be the only way of obtaining sexual satisfaction. Other forms of communication were recognized as being equally important by the disabled group (see Figure 5.16). These included talking to, smelling and touching your partner. While 58% of the SB/HC group felt that they knew how to excite their partner (see Figure 5.17), 60% of the same group stated that urinary incontinence (both in terms of explana-

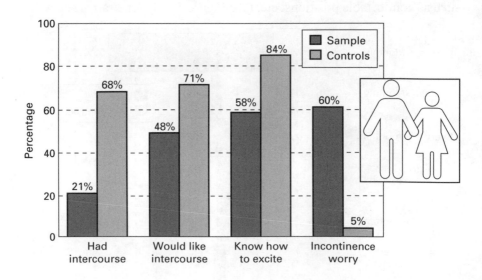

Figure 5.15 Sexual relationships

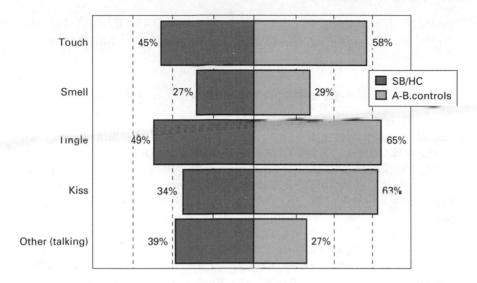

Figure 5.16 Communicating with partner

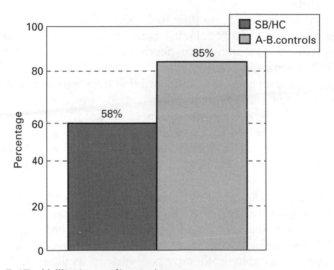

Figure 5.17 Ability to excite partner

tion and management) was the greatest problem and barrier to overcome in a sexual relationship (see Figure 5.15). Six disabled adults requested specific information about catheter management, ten about urinary leakage, six about positioning the catheter during love-making and thirteen about positions for love-making. Clearly, continence was not a concern for the able-bodied control group. In an open-ended question at the end of the section, nineteen of the SB/HC group thought that changing society's attitude towards the sexuality of disabled people was essential. If this could be achieved, those with SB/HC thought that this might improve the overall availability and quality of information for disabled people.

Analysis of the structured interviews – Key issues

Over the last two decades there has been an increasing interest in the sexual problems and preoccupations of people with disabilities, but particularly those with SB/HC (Anderson and Clarke 1982, Blackburn *et al.* 1991, Blackburn and Bax 1992, Cass *et al.* 1986, Dorner 1977, 1980, 1990, Edser and Ward 1991, Sloan 1991). The complications of neurological, physiological and cognitive impairment often associated with this population may be further compounded by the psychological and social concerns related to their sexual interests, function and activity (Dorner 1977). A need for appropriate sex education and counselling for adults with SB/HC, which continues throughout life, has been identified within this study. Improvement in sex education curriculum for able-bodied people is also acknowledged and considered necessary.

Sex education

Although 80% of the SB/HC sample had received sex education at some stage of their lives (see Figure 5.1), information was not always consistent and appropriate to their individual needs or their complex disabilities. Many of these young adults complained that texts/information were often too long, written in an academic style and that diagrams and illustrations frequently depicted stereotypical 'able-bodied, white, body beautiful' male and female images, with whom they could not identify. Illustrations seldom showed people wearing a stoma bag, a penile urinal appliance, with a catheter in situ or information on how to deal with bowels in a sexual relationship. ASBAH, SPOD, the Brook Advisory and The Ann Craft Trust (formerly NAPSAC) all design materials specifically for disabled people and have sought to reform the image of 'white, able-bodied' sex education materials. Many of the disabled adults complained that their sex education was segregated from able-bodied programmes. Two men in the SB/HC group were told that they could leave the sex education class and attend the hydrotherapy pool instead, as the material would be irrelevant to them!

The sample who had received adult sex education might be seen as advocates promoting the continuation of sex education throughout adultlife. Although the importance of early sex education, socialization and interaction cannot be over-emphasized, sexual awareness and attraction for most people continues throughout life (Sloan 1991). This suggests that sex education, although important throughout childhood and adolescence may need to continue, particularly for those with complex disabilities, during adult life. Many teenagers with SB/HC have infrequent opportunities to socialize with their peers, often being isolated outside of school and preferring to mix with able-bodied people rather than their disabled peers (Edser and Ward 1991, Thomas *et al.* 1989). This study suggests that an increasing number of disabled adults want to know about their sexuality, are engaging in sexual relationships, and requesting appropriate information and sexual counselling beyond adolescence. Three members of the SB/HC sample had displayed 'inappropriate sexual behaviour' in public, e.g. masturbation, and in consequence had received some counselling support.

Many of these adults were only prepared, or were given the opportunity, to discuss sexuality for the first time. In contrast, the 59 young disabled adults age 18–25 years who were interviewed about sexuality in the Thomas *et al.*'s (1989) study, welcomed an earlier opportunity to discuss sexual matters with someone they trusted. Their sample included young adults with spina bifida, cerebral palsy and other disabilities who may have felt comfortable discussing sexual matters at an earlier age. Eighty per cent of the young disabled adults in this study stated that the author was the first person with whom they had discussed sexual concerns; such as sexual relationships, love-making and continence management, genetic risks, masturbation, wet dreams and erections. The Warnock report (1978) indicated that sex education and counselling provision for disabled people was particularly poor in schools, with limited information being provided about individual disabilities. This study has suggested that both teaching and explanation of terms (such as areas of the anatomy and activities such as masturbation) should be provided at times to suit the individual's cognitive ability, chronological age and individual needs. Positive attitudes towards the teaching of sex can and should be fostered in schools so that information can be presented in the context of loving and meaningful relationships as well as family life (Edser and Ward, 1991). In consequence, some disabled people may feel more comfortable discussing sex, and others may be discouraged from displaying inappropriate sexual behaviour in public places. The Education Acts have recommended the inclusion of sex education curriculum in all schools; sex education should 'have due regard to moral considerations and the value of family life' (Education Act 1996). Personal and Social Health Education curriculum should encompass the moral, religious and cultural beliefs of the individual. Disabled people should never be 'put down' and their particular individual sexual needs, within the cultural ethos of their disability, should not be overlooked.

Puberty and precocious puberty
Precocious or advanced puberty means the early or late onset of puberty. This has been described as 'the most frequent endocrine manifestation of children treated for non-tumoral hydrocephalus' (Brauner *et al.* 1991). In her review of the international literature of the onset of pubertal development in myelomeningocele, Furman (1990) noted that the incidence of precocious puberty in this population was between 4.42 and 5.8%.

Thirteen per cent of this study sample reported an onset of puberty between 7 and 10 years, with 5% reporting having regular periods from the same age. Two women had their first period at 6 years of age. By comparison, four teenagers had menstruated regularly before they were 11 years old and seven reported irregular periods (Dorner 1977). Nineteen per cent of the females with SB/HC reported irregular periods at less than two-monthly intervals with many reporting mood swings and feelings of irritability occurring either just before or at the beginning of menstruation. The disabled women were concerned that irregular menses might minimize their chances of conception. In my 'observational diaries' I had noted that five women (5%) whose periods occurred at less than six-monthly intervals were over 23 years of age. These women already showed physical signs of premature ageing. These features included the presence of grey hair, some wrinkles and fine lines and hirsutism. Although it is difficult to postulate about the possible correlation between precocious puberty and premature ageing, further research is indicated to examine the average age of onset of puberty and assess the true incidence of precocious puberty, as well as examine any possible links between precocious puberty and premature ageing. Current available data on the true incidence of precocious puberty within this population is limited and includes Brauner *et al.* (1991) and Furman (1990). Recent advances in technology mean that a larger number of people with SB/HC are surviving into adulthood (Blum *et al.* 1991), and are therefore presenting with additional sexual concerns which warrant well-informed discussion and appropriate advice.

Continence and sexuality

Both urinary and bowel incontinence were two of the most significant documented findings within this study. Sixty per cent of the young disabled adults expressed concerns about urinary continence and sexuality. Of these, 28% expressed particular concern about their 'bowels and sexuality issues'. Although six adults stated that the smell of urine was 'off putting' for some partners with whom they were having a relationship, three adults were unaware of their odours and oblivious that their smell might offend their partners. Those adults who had experienced intimate sex, elaborated on some of the personal difficulties that they had encountered concerning continence. These included discussing continence with their partners, carers and professionals. In particular, they found it difficult to discuss how to make continence more aesthetically pleasing, the lack of and availability of information, specific methods and techniques for handling incontinence. Castree and Walker (1981), Dorner (1977), and Thomas *et al.* (1989) also reported similar concerns addressing sexuality and continence.

Where necessary, and with the young person's consent, I made referrals to the ASBAH counselling/or Disabled Living Advisory service for advice and information. Regrettably, the ASBAH counselling service was devolved during the study, necessitating referral routes to other counselling agencies.

Sexual function

Research regarding the sexual function of people with SB/HC has been relatively limited. Cass and colleagues (1986) reported that satisfactory sexual function was commonest in those young adults with SB/HC with lesions below the Sacralone level. This study highlighted innumerable questions about the young person's concerns regarding their sexual function. Twenty-three per cent of young men with SB/HC reported that they had erections with several men commenting that their erections had ceased after 16 years of age.

Qualitative results – Key issues

This section focuses principally on the SB/HC group's research findings. Diary observation data is included here, in addition to the qualitative information, particularly where consent had been refused to tape record interviews but given for note-taking. Information was requested from the ABC group regarding the following definitions: 'friendship', 'love', 'relationship' and 'sex.' The data obtained to date indicated that some of the disabled people had difficulty in offering some explanation of these four terms.

A wealth of information from the SB/HC sample was gathered for this small study. Only the significant findings will be reported here. Information which was repeated by the SB/HC group in the structured interviews is not discussed again here. Of the sixteen adults with SB/HC, there were nine females and seven males.

Four of the SB/HC adults lived with parents, four lived independently and not with a partner, one man lived with his wife at home, another lived with his wife in residential care, one woman lived with her fiance and parents, while three lived alone with parents and two lived in residential accommodation. One of the able-bodied controls had a visual disability. No other disabilities were reported among the able-bodied group. All the controls were unmarried, twelve lived at home and three were sharing accommodation with friends. All of the able-bodied young people reported that they were having a relationship. None of the able-bodied young people had children.

General comments

Four of the SB/HC group felt uneasy discussing sex and spoke about other issues, such as independence training. I did not force them to discuss sexuality. I was much more concerned that they felt at ease with the interview. However, they were happy to answer the four questions concerning friendship, love, etc. (Appendix 5). The control responses were generally factual and precise and they provided definitions of the following terms: friendship, love, relationships and sex.

Marital status

Two of the SB/HC males were married and three females were engaged. Two of the engaged women have since married. None of the SB/HC group had children at the time of interview, although some of the young disabled adults have since had children.

Terminology

Seventeen of the SB/HC adults agreed to discuss terminology associated with bodily functions, puberty and sexuality set out below. In some instances, respondents gave more than one answer to particular questions, while in others they declined to give a response at all, i.e. for the sexual intercourse question. There was a richness both in the variety and quality of responses received. Although some of the responses may appear humorous, they were not intended to provoke such a response. They were said with frankness and honesty and highlighted the paucity of information available about sex and sexuality available for disabled people.

Of particular note were comments about the following: 'period' 'virgin', 'what sperm looks like?', 'what is masturbation?', 'what is sexual intercourse?'. The following responses were provided.

Description of 'period: menstruation'

- Two answered 'yes' only.
- Three spoke of eggs retreating from the ovaries but did not define the outcome.
- Four spoke specifically of monthly bleeding.
- One thought blood came from the vagina.
- Three 'knew there was blood' but 'could not describe where the blood came from'.
- Two defined period as 'a female maturing'.

Description of 'virgin'

- Two thought it was 'a non-meat eater'.
- Thirteen thought it was 'someone who had not had sex' (usually a woman).
- Four thought it related to women only.
- Two had never heard of the term.

Description of 'sperm'

- Four said it resembled 'a tadpole'.
- One described it as 'frog-spawn'.
- Nine described it as 'a creamy, whitish fluid'.
- Two stated that 'a microscope was required to see it'.
- Two could not respond.

Description of 'masturbation'

- Two adults defined it as 'self abuse'.
- One adult described it as 'playing with yourself'.
- One adult described it as 'yes...umhh...'.
- Four adults described it as 'stimulating your sexual organs ... both men and women do it'.
- Four adults described it as 'rubbing the penis up and down'.
- One adult thought it was 'an orgasm'.
- Two adults thought it was 'producing sperm'.
- One adult suggested it was 'when a man has sexual urges normally to the opposite sex'.

Description of 'sexual intercourse'

- Two men described it as 'mating'.
- Two men 'as pumping the woman'.
- One man as 'fucking a woman'.
- One woman stated it was 'something to do when intent on reproduction'.
- Three adults described it as 'sex'.
- Two adults defined it as 'reproduction'.
- One adult described it as 'a man starts to get excited and the woman ... uuuhhh'.
- One adult described it as 'when a man and woman take part in sex, this is where a man's penis is put in the lady's virginia and a certain position is taken up'.
- Three 'could not' as opposed to 'refused' to answer the question.
- Two did not wish to answer the question.

Sexual experiences

With the exception of two men and two women, 12 of the SB/HC group were currently in, or had previously had, a relationship. One woman was ambivalent about her sexual preferences. Two men were homosexual and two men reported bisexual feelings. One of the bisexual men openly described some of his feelings 'There was this big man just lying there on all fours, of course me being in Paradise...' He also referred to his guilt and ambivalence about being bi-sexual. He claimed that his marriage had not been consummated and he could only enjoy sex with his homosexual partner. He still enjoyed his wife's social company and her emotional support.

All 17 of the SB/HC sample wished to have a relationship, although full penetrative sex was not necessarily regarded as 'an essential ingredient' (stated one male respondent).

Continence

Six expressed particular concerns about explaining and managing urinary and bowel continence to their partner(s): 'I knew I smelt' was one response, 'How do I explain the bag... catheters?' (2), and 'Can I make love with a catheter in place?'(4).

Wet dreams

Two women and two men thought wet dreams referred to their urinary incontinence.

Abuse

Ten of the SB/HC group retrospectively disclosed physical, sexual or emotional abuse. At the time of the interviews two adults were still being abused. One female control disclosed physical abuse. All were appropriately followed up by the local social service and health departments to ensure that they were protected from further harm and offered counselling support.

Loving definitions

Sixteen of the SB/HC group and fifteen of the ABC participants offered individual explanations for friendship, relationships, love and sex. All sixteen SB/HC individuals gave verbal answers. Nine of the SB/HC individuals preferred discussing the terms rather than writing them down. Forming letters and holding a pen were reported to be particularly difficult tasks. In their study of hand function in children with myelomeningocele, Mazur and colleagues (1988) noted that children with low intelligence (IQ <80) and those with high lesions experienced difficulty using their hands, particularly hand-writing skills. The ABC group preferred writing to discussing these questions. The ABC group felt that they would be able to answer more honestly and feel less embarrassed.

Friendship

Sixteen SB/HC adults (nine females and seven males) all answered this question compared with eleven controls. The collated responses suggest that 'friendship' encompasses features shown in Table 5.2.

All respondents thought that friendship was not specifically related to the gender issue, usually involved two or more people, and did not include penetrative sex. One male and one female with SB/HC summarized friendship as follows:

Table 5.2 The features thought to characterize friendship

	SB/HC (*n*)	Control (*n*)
Trust	7	4
Confide	8	3
Caring/hoping	4	3
Fun	5	1
Talking	7	1
Unity	2	1
Understanding	1	1
Enjoyment	1	1
Loyalty	1	1
Relate to someone	2	2
Two or more people	3	3

SB/HC, *n* = 16; controls, *n* = 11; four non-respondents.

Male with SB/HC

This is a relationship in which people are able to confide in one another, have fun and care for one another, but are not emotionally involved with one another. (The word *emotional* in this interview seemed to relate to a sexual relationship.)

Female with SB/HC

Friendship to me is having a friend you can trust and have a laugh with and someone you can confide in; that to me is what a friendship is all about.

Relationships

All sixteen adults with SB/HC answered this questions compared with ten of the controls. Two individuals from the SB/HC group described a relationship as a mixture of 'friendship and love' and being 'one step on from a relationship'. One adult control described it as either 'sexual can be platonic'. The features thought to characterize relationships are shown in Table 5.3.

Table 5.3 The features thought to characterize relationships

	SB/HC (*n*)	Control (*n*)
Trust	4	0
Caring	4	0
Sharing experiences	2	1
May include sex	5	2
May exclude sex	4	3
Very close friends	5	2

SB/HC, *n* = 16; controls, *n* = 13; two non-respondents

Love

All sixteeen of the SB/HC group offered definitions compared with eleven of the controls. There was some overlap in relation to the explanations offered for friendship and love. The author feels that the following statement by a young woman with SB/HC summarizes many of the contributors definitions of 'love':

> Love is a very strong word, you can't just fall in and out of love. Love is being involved and a bit like friendship but much stronger, feeling of being safe with the person that you love.

Although I recognize that further research may need to be undertaken addressing some of the definitions, these initial results suggested that love may include the features shown in Table 5.4.

Table 5.4 The features thought to characterize love

	SB/HC (*n*)	Control (*n*)
Trust	4	1
Caring	4	1
Sharing experiences	1	1
Love for parents	3	2
Love for partner	3	2
Love for someone	7	4
Hugs/kisses/intercourse	Na	Na
May exclude sex	4	3
Very close friends	5	2
Deep affection		
Reciprocity	3	1

SB/HC, *n* = 16; controls, *n* = 13; two non-respondents; Na = not answered.

Sex

Sixteen of the SB/HC group and ten of the ABC group volunteered definitions of sex. Some of the interpretations are listed in Table 5.5.

Table 5.5 The features thought to characterize sex

	SB/HC (*n*)	Control (*n*)
Sharing experiences	1	1
Love for someone	3	2
Intercourse	11	4
Physical contact with/without sex	3	3
Love for partner	3	2
Love for someone	7	4
Having a baby	1	2

SB/HC, *n* – 16; controls, *n* = 10; five non-respondents.

Discussion

The cocktail party syndrome (CPS)

Hadenius *et al.* (1962) (cited in Tew 1991) first used this term to describe the behaviour of some people with hydrocephalus who displayed 'a peculiar contrast between a good ability to learn words and talk and not knowing what they talk about. They love to chatter but think illogically'. This occurs in about 25–30% of adults with SB/HC (Thomas *et al.* 1989). People with this condition have been described as 'chatterers or blatherers', who display unusual verbal fluency but notable cognitive weaknesses, particularly in relation to their reasoning and perceptions of situations.

Tew (1991) noted that cocktail party syndrome (CPS) is not a particular feature of those with spina bifida, nor necessarily of poor intellect, nor indeed everybody who has hydrocephalus. It is a feature of some people with HC. Tew (1979) used five criteria to identify people with CPS and Hurley *et al.* (1990) also suggested that each person must have at least four of these criteria. These included:

1. The excessive use of phrases in conversation.
2. Inappropriate and irrelevant contexts of conversations.
3. Fluent, well-articulated speech.
4. Overfamiliarity.
5. Variation of responses.

The three adults who displayed CPS behaviour in this study all had HC in addition to SB. Three revealed at least four of Tew's four of the aforementioned CPS criteria, particularly criteria 1, 2 and 4. Arguably some of the topics and ensuing responses discussed with the author may have been prompted by the subject matter. If researchers discuss sex with disabled people, they must anticipate that some people may feel uninhibited and speak more frankly about this subject than others. Equally, the disabled person may be extremely anxious about some of the questions being asked and display 'inappropriate and irrelevant chatter' to overcome his/her shyness or embarrassment. Some people initiated other discussion topics in order to avoid discussing 'sex' and I was particularly careful not to develop the discussion if the disabled person felt at all anxious. Once the three more 'chatty' individuals focused their conversation, they seemed happy to discuss their most intimate experiences. Three people with SB/HC were especially shy. Some conversations were initiated and developed by myself but carefully monitored to avoid any embarrassment. This suggests that not all adults display or necessarily conform to Tew's CPS criteria. Although the precise cause of CPS still remains unclear, some researchers have favoured a neuro-pathological explanation of this behaviour (Tew 1991). Cocktail party syndrome seems to occur less frequently in young children (Tew 1991).

Three of the disabled group interviewed required assistance in focusing their discussions. They were garrulous and 'chatted' about a variety of unrelated issues, sometimes inappropriately and occasionally needed assistance in focusing their thoughts. One man could have spoken uninterruptedly for several hours about 'sheltered workshops', the financial exploitation of disabled people as well as his sexuality. After several minutes, I felt obliged to intervene, refocus his thoughts and we agreed to conclude the interview within a defined time-scale.

Terminology

There was some comparison between some of the interpretations of friendship, relationship and love offered by both the SB/HC and ABC groups: trust, sharing and confidence being described as some of the necessary features by the SB/HC group. 'Sex' for eleven of the SB/HC group implied 'penetrative intercourse', although five of the same group acknowledged that 'sex' could be communicated and reciprocated in other ways, such as loving, touching, petting, 'sharing your body meaningfully with someone'. Thomas *et al.* (1989) noted that 'genuine friendships' had other interpretations. They were not necessarily attributed to grandparents, health professionals, day-centre staff or taxi drivers, but by the degree of 'closeness' with that particular person. Relationships in their study implied 'special friends' or someone with whom the young person could adopt a 'counselling and understanding role'. Friendships which are often regarded as superficial by a socially active able-bodied adolescent may be considered 'best' friends by the inexperienced teenager with spina bifida and hydrocephalus (Edser and Ward, 1991). Whether the terms have individual or broad definitions, the significant issue is that they are explained and understood by the disabled person.

Abuse

The literature challenges and refutes the previous notion that disabled children and adults cannot be abused (see Marchant 1991, Westcott 1993). The incidence of reported abuse varies in the literature (Blackburn 1995). Several factors may contribute to these variations:

- The purpose and nature of the study and what information it is trying to elucidate.
- The type and severity of disability.
- The gender and age of the interviewee.
- Ethnicity.
- Specific criteria and definitions of abuse being applied.

Recordings of prevalence or incidence of abuse within England and Wales used to be inconsistent (Westcott 1993). Reliable figures depend on child care agencies having access to, and the resources to record and disseminate, such information consistently. Such information is now recorded by all local authorities in England and Wales and submitted to the Department of Health, Social Care Department, along with other information, such as the nature of the abuse, gender and age distribution.

However, this study was primarily aimed to elicit information about sexual knowledge and experiences and not specifically abuse. Retrospective abuse was disclosed during the qualitative interviews only (physical, sexual, emotional and neglect). The structured interviews did not include questions addressing the physical, emotional and sexual 'abuse' of disabled adults. I believe abuse disclosure might have been higher than the 10% reported had the structured interviews also incorporated questions about abuse.

Turk and Brown (1992) examined the incidence and nature of sexual abuse in a group of adults with learning difficulties. They reported that 23% of the women had experienced 'non-contact' sexual abuse (e.g. indecent exposure) and over 90% contact (physical) abuse. The incidence of abuse may be deemed to be higher in those studies which specifically seek to obtain such information. Any abuse, in whatever form but particularly involving disabled people, is a serious concern and a violation of their human rights. Abuse for the disabled person may have a much broader definition. The Children Act (DoH, 1991c) states 'that a person with a disability qualifies for services before and after the age of 18 years'.

Most children by 18 years of age are considered adults and can legally choose and make most decisions independently, i.e. without another adult's authority. The Act offers no recommendations for more vulnerable adults who have attained the chronological age of majority (18 years) but who may be younger in terms of their social and emotional maturity. The mean average age of the SB/HC group in this study was 23.5 years and indicated the vulnerability of some of these young adults. Some of these adults may require services and protection from abuse well after attaining 18 years of age. The Department of Health (2000) recognizes that there could be 'no hiding places' when it came to exposing the abuse of disabled adults. In their guidance, the Department stresses the importance of protecting victims and witnesses and describes an inter-agency framework and procedures for responding to individual cases of abuse.

Denying disabled adults the right to sexual fulfilment, independence and choice may increase their poor self image and esteem, and make them more vulnerable to abuse (Thomas *et al.* 1989). Until recently, society was often 'retarded' in accepting the physical and emotional needs and the contribution of disabled people and their need for autonomy but protection from harm (Blackburn, 1995).

Cognitive assessments

The pilot samples were not equally matched for IQ because of the difficulty in tracing previous, reliable IQ recordings from this particular disabled population. This must, therefore, have implications for how the information is interpreted. Even when matched for IQs, specific patterns may not necessarily emerge. Other factors such as aetiology, educational attainment, environment, general physical health and individual medical history (that is the numbers of shunt blockages and infections) should not be ignored. Three of the disabled people who were living at home had received more formal education. They attained higher test scores on assessment than those living in residential care. Three of the sample demonstrated significantly higher verbal than performance abilities. This suggests that this population may have difficulty with non-verbal reasoning and thinking and may relate better to visual images. This could have implications on how materials are both designed and presented within the learning environment.

Of the seven SB/HC adults who completed the cognitive assessments, four of them had taken part in both the qualitative and quantitative interviews (total pilot sample, $n=8$). The following tests were performed and recorded by a psychologist: Wechsler Adult Intelligence Scale revised tests (WAIS-R) classified two people of average intelligence, three with minor learning difficulties and two with moderate to severe learning difficulties ($n=7$) (see Appendix 8). On verbal-performance differences, using scaled scores by age for each adult, three people showed significant verbal performance differences ($P<0.05$), with the verbal IQ being significantly higher than the performance IQ. Seven individuals completed WAIS verbal (digit span, vocabulary, arithmetic, comprehension similarities) tests. Performance sub-tests included arranging and completing pictures, block assembling and designing blocks. Only one person performed above the 75th percentile (reflecting strengths in comparison to individuals of similar age). Four fell below the 25th percentile reflecting weaknesses compared to the performance of other individuals of the same age.

One lady was too shy to complete all of the tests. Her results are therefore excluded here. The mean average age of the sub-sample was 24.2 years.

6 Sex and the law

Introduction

This chapter does not intend to provide a legal guide to sexual behaviour but rather an *aide-memoire* for those staff who may wish to differentiate between both criminal and civil law. Both are briefly addressed in this chapter and in Appendix 6. Criminal law is the conduct prohibited by law, and civil law addresses the regulation of disputes over the rights and obligations of persons dealing with each.

The law relevant to sexual behaviour is often an area of great uncertainty and concern for professionals, parents and young disabled people alike. The chapter specifically addresses negligence, the duty of care, consent and some of the sexuality and disability legal concerns that health professionals may encounter during their work.

Many staff caring for disabled adults are often unaware, fear or do not understand the law. This often increases apprehension in relation to managing sensitive issues (Gunn 1996). This might include advising a young disabled person about 'continence' management before sex. Furthermore, parents/carers sometimes have difficulty in accepting their disabled son or daughter as a person with sexual feelings and do not always recognize their son's or daughter's need for sexual fulfilment. This is largely because of society's previously mentioned attitudes, reservations and prejudices about disabled people having sex on religious or moral grounds. As noted in Chapter 4, several parents feared that their son or daughter might display inappropriate sexual behaviour in public, such as masturbating in the street, a residential unit or a classroom. Although some parents acknowledged that masturbation was a natural and normal feature of sexuality, they were fearful of the consequences of inappropriate displays of sexual behaviour by their sons and daughters in public places, which might lead to police investigation. They recognized that this could be further complicated if the disabled person had communication difficulties and no appropriate intermediary or interpreter present at the time of the incident to support or advise them.

The civil law

In civil matters there is no concept of punishment. In civil matters, a case must be proved *on the balance of probability*. In criminal proceedings, the prosecution must prove its case *beyond reasonable doubt.* People guilty of crimes are usually punished by fines, community services or imprisonment.

Sex and the law – a civil perspective

The United Nations Declaration on the Rights of Mentally Retarded Persons[1] stated that 'people with learning difficulties have the same basic rights as other people of that same country and same age'. This does not include a particular right to sexual fulfilment. Currently there is no law enshrining the right to sexuality, although the Human Rights Act 1998, addressed in more detail below, may now provide some legal challenges, particularly under Articles 12 and 14 (the right to marry and have a family and the right to prohibition against discrimination). While it is recognized that disabled people should be able to explore their sexual needs, this has to be balanced with the need to protect vulnerable people who may risk being abused.

Human Rights Act 1998

In October 2000, the Human Rights Act 1998 was introduced into England and Wales. This Act is based on the European Convention of Human Rights legislation and gives further effect to the rights and freedoms guaranteed under the European Convention. The Act is not specifically related to disability but may impact on some of the laws related to disabled people, such as the Disability Discrimination Act 1995. The principal Articles of the Human Rights Act that are most likely to impact on disabled people are:

- Article 2 – The right to life.
- Article 3 – Freedom from torture or inhuman or degrading treatment or punishment.
- Article 8 – The right to respect for privacy and family life.
- Article 10 – The right to freedom of expression.
- Article 12 – The right to marry and have a family.
- Article 14 – Prohibition of discrimination.

All these articles confer absolute rights. A list of other articles is included in Appendix 6. Section 6 of the Human Rights Act 1998 imposes a duty on public authorities to act compatibly with the European Convention on Human Rights, subject to specified exceptions[2]. NHS Trusts and other

---

[1] UN Department of Social Affairs 1971, New York.

[2] Not unlawful for a public authority to act in a way which is incompatible with a Convention Right if (a) as the result of one or more provisions of primary legislation, the authority could not have acted differently, or (b) in the case of one or more provisions of, or made under, primary legislation which cannot be read or given effect in a way which is compatible with the Convention Rights, the authority was acting so as to give effect to or enforce those provisions s6(2) of the Human Rights Act 1998.

NHS organizations are classified as public authorities under section 6 of the Act. This means that these bodies have a duty to act in agreement with the law. At present, a doctor caring for an NHS patient will be acting under a 'public authority' but not when he or she treats private patients in a private hospital[3] for a professional fee.

Article 2 Human Rights Act 1998

The courts now have to consider the duty imposed in Article 2 – the right to life – and the duty imposed by the domestic law of negligence. If an NHS organization is obliged to make adequate provision for medical care and fails to do so in circumstances where either death ensues or where injury is sustained in circumstances where there was a real and immediate risk to life, there may be a breach of Article 2.

The fundamental nature of the right to life was acknowledged as 'the most fundamental of human rights' and called for 'the most anxious scrutiny' *Buddaycay v. Secretary of State for the Home Department {1987} AC 514 at 531G*. Until recently, the right to life had largely been unexplored by the English domestic courts, with the exception of the leading case of Airedale NHS Trust vs Bland *Airedale NHS Trust v. Bland {1993} AC 78, the case of Tony Bland* and the recent High Court decision in the case of Ms B. (2002). The courts may in future be confronted with imaginative and progressive arguments as people begin to test the boundaries to the right to life.

It follows from the Commission's decision in *X v. UK 1978 14 DR at 33* that the state must take 'adequate and appropriate steps to protect life'. Domestic courts could face the argument that Primary Care Trusts and NHS Acute Trusts are obliged to make 'adequate and appropriate' provision for medical care in all those cases where the right to life of a patient could otherwise be endangered. A right to life may also extend to cases where injury has occurred and there is a real and immediate risk to life *Osman v. UK {1999} 5 BHRC 293*.

If the domestic courts find the obligations imposed by Article 2 more onerous than the Common Law duty of care, then the scope for liability on the part of NHS Trusts and Primary Care Trusts could be increased.

Article 3

Article 3 states that 'no one shall be subjected to torture or degrading treatment or punishment'. The European Commission has held that medical treatment of an experimental character and without the consent of the person involved may in some circumstances be prohibited by Article 3 as demonstrated in the case of *X v. Denmark {1983} 32 DR 282*. Here medical treatment of an experimental nature and without the consent of the person involved was regarded as a breach of Article 3. Treatment of an experimental nature could mean treatment which is not yet properly

---

[3] See 583 HL Official Report (5th series) col 811 9, 24 November 1997.

established. This could have implications for new treatments which are being considered or trialled.

Article 8

Article 8 of the Human Rights Act 1998 guarantees 'an individual's right to respect for his private family and family life, his home and correspondence'. An individual's medical records forms an intimate part of his or her private life. The disclosure of such records, particularly about an individual's sexual activity, unless it can be justified on account of sexual abuse could constitute a breach of that article.

Negligence

All health professionals owe a duty of care to their patients. This duty of care requires health care practitioners to act in a reasonable manner to the standard of another similarly qualified professional and to protect their patients from 'harm'. As a general rule, if a professional acts in accordance with the common practice of other similar professionals, he or she would not be negligent. However, the practice or procedure itself *might* be perceived as negligent (*Roberge v. Bolduc {1991} 78DLR*). Where a person holds him or herself out as having a specialist skill, such as a urologist or continence adviser, he or she will be judged on by the objective standards of a reasonably competent person exercising that skill.

The *Bolam Test* has been described as what a responsible body of peers would do in the circumstances; in this case this might be other continence and/or sexual health advisers. *Bolam* suggested that a health professional, such as a doctor, was not negligent when acting in accordance with recognized practice. The *Bolam Test* has survived a number of legal challenges over the last few years[4].

A real challenge presents when the health professional is particularly experienced and practises in a highly specialized field. Should that person exercise *greater* care than the ordinary competent professional? Although not easy to answer, the case of *Maynard v. West Midlands Regional Health Authority {1984}* stated that 'a doctor who professes to exercise a special skill must exercise the ordinary skill of his speciality'.

Duty of care

Establishing a duty of care is not usually a major problem in health care cases where patients/clients are in hospital. In such circumstances, health care staff are clearly responsible for their care. In general practice or in the community, health professionals owe a duty of care to the patients/clients they look after or who are on their lists or are known to them.

It is more difficult to establish when health professionals are responsible for people who are not on their lists or not known to them. The legal test for the extent of duties of care in negligence may be divided into two parts.

---

[4] *Bolitho v. City & Hackney HA {1998} AC 232: Sidaway v. Governors of Bethlem Royal Hospital {1985} AC 871.*

The first is to ascertain whether it is foreseeable that the patient could be affected by the health professional's actions. For example, if health professionals could anticipate what might happen to their patients, then they may owe a duty of care towards those patients). The second is to assess whether the duty of care is 'just and reasonable'. For example, doctors giving contraceptive advice do not owe a duty of care to future sexual partners of their patients as was highlighted in the case of *Goodwill v. British Pregnancy Advisory Service {1996} 2 ALL ER 161*. Disabled people of any age should receive appropriate information, advice and support about treatments and management that might seem controversial. If a patient is negligently discharged from hospital or care while still infectious, then a duty of care would be owed to others who might in consequence be infected.

There is generally no legal obligation to help victims of an accident merely because they might benefit from assistance. However, a district nurse or health visitor might be obliged by their contracts of their employment to stop and care for an accident victim (Montgomery 1997). If a continence advisor advises or counsels a patient about managing their urinary incontinence during a sexual relationship, not only should the advisor be competent to advise on such matters but the duty of care should extend to advising the client and minimizing any possible exploitation or harm. This could involve teaching patients how to deal with their own sexuality, for example the management of incontinence, but could also include information on how to deal with sexual approaches from others.

Principles of patient confidentiality

All NHS organizations have a Common Law duty of confidentiality. Personal information about patients held by health professionals is subject to a legal duty of confidence and should not be disclosed without the consent of the person. Imparting any information without the consent of the individual would be a breach of confidence.

Confidentiality should only be broken in exceptional circumstances and only after very careful consideration that such a breach can be justified. The categories where a breach of confidence may be justified include:

- Giving evidence in court.
- Statements made in the paramount interests of a child to legitimate inquirers.
- The public interest.

The courts normally balance the public interests favouring confidentiality against those advising disclosure in the particular circumstances of each case. The question remains one for the courts and not for professional bodies (Kennedy and Grubb 1998). The legal obligations imposed upon healthcare professionals who deal with confidential information supplied to them by patients is now largely codified by statute.

The Data Protection Act 1998 came into force in March 2000 and implemented the 1995 European Community Data Protection Directive. The use of personal information held on manual as well as computer records is now governed by law. The Common Law duty of confidence applies to personal data provided in confidence by patients. This must be complied with to meet the first principle of the Data Protection Act 1998, which requires fair and lawful processing of information. The Data Protection Act 1998 does not itself prevent NHS organizations from using personal data for legitimate medical purposes, which *may* include the management of healthcare services[5].

The Health Service Circular HSC 2000/009: *Data Protection Act 1998: Protection and Use of Patient Information* (published on 23 March 2000) highlights the main implications for the NHS of the Data Protection Act 1998, associated Orders and Regulations and the actions that NHS Trusts must take in order to comply with the new legislation. The above Health Service Circular stresses the following:

- All staff dealing with personal information must comply with the Data Protection Act 1998 and associated provisions, in particular those concerning the rights of data subjects (patients) in respect of access to and use of information in their health records.
- All staff dealing with personal information must be aware of the requirements of the Common Law duty of confidence. Any negotiations with a third party to process personal data on behalf of the organization must be subject to a written contract, which requires compliance with appropriate security and confidentiality arrangements.

The case of *W v. Egdell {1990} 2WLR 47* concerned W, who had been convicted of manslaughter after multiple killings in circumstances of extreme violence. W was detained under the Mental Health Act 1983 as a patient within a secure hospital. Dr Egdell was instructed by solicitors on behalf of W to prepare a psychiatric report. Dr Egdell believed that the contents of his report were of public interest as the report contained information regarding W's dangerous behaviour and should be disclosed to the medical director caring for W as well as to the Home Office, to ensure that the public were not endangered by W's possible early release from prison. The public interest in protecting the public from harm took precedence over the general public interest in ensuring the confidentiality of the medical consultation.

Confidentiality – key points

- All health professionals are under an overriding ethical as well as a legal duty to protect the health and safety of their patients.
- NHS organizations should ensure that local procedures are in place relating to confidentiality and setting out the principles governing the

---

[5] The Data Protection (Subject Access Modification) (Health) Order 2000.

appropriate sharing of information, as per the Health Service Circular HSC 2000/009: Data Protection Act 1998.

- In certain circumstances, it may be necessary to disclose or exchange personal information about an individual. This will need to be in accordance with the Data Protection Act 1998.
- Article 8 of the Human Rights Act 1998 preserves an individual's right to respect for his private family and family life, his home and correspondence. An individual's medical records forms an intimate part of his or her private life. The disclosure of such records, unless it can be justified with reference to Article 8(2), will constitute a breach of Article 8. Examples where disclosure was justified in the interests of public health include the case of *TV v. Finland {1994} 76-a-DR 140 Ecom HR*.

Criminal law

There are a number of specific offences which are punishable by the criminal courts in relation to sexual activity. The criminal law can be divided into two areas: (a) general illegal activities that affect all individuals, and (b) specific offences when one of the parties involved may be a 'vulnerable' person. Criminal Court proceedings are normally open to the public. In 1985 the Crown Prosecution Service was set up under the Director of Public Prosecutions (DPP). Each region has its own Chief Crown Prosecutor who has the powers to prosecute serious offences. The main Act in England and Wales prohibiting certain activities related to sexual activity is set out in the Sexual Offences Act 1956 and its various amendments (see Appendix 6). This is still the major legislation in England and Wales which condemns non-consensual sexual intercourse. Sexual intercourse is defined as penetration by the man's penis (s44 Sexual Offences Act 1956). However, penile penetration may not always necessarily include penile ejaculation.

The purpose of legislation prohibiting various sexual activities is to prevent exploitation and the sexual abuse of individuals. The original Sexual Offences Act 1956:

1. Defines the criminal activity.
2. Defines the situations in which the criminal act occurs.
3. Outlines the sanctions that apply whenever a specific crime occurs.

Aiding and abetting

A health professional might be perceived of aiding and abetting a criminal activity if, for example, that health professional assisted two people to have sexual intercourse, and the female had severe learning difficulties. This is on the basis that 'a mentally defective woman', within the Sexual Offences Act, would be unable to consent to sexual intercourse. Where there is a policy within NHS Trusts which permits private accommodation for women with capacity to conduct sexual activity with privacy and dignity, it is less likely, although not entirely impossible, that grounds for criminal activity could take place. Health professionals working in this speciality fully comprehend the limits imposed on their practice by the law. Child protection and disability teams often seek the opinions of specialists when a young disabled person has been arrested for alleged indecent behaviour and inappropriate touching. The fundamental problem often lies with the young person being unable to relieve or deal with his or her sexual frustration in a private place. However, teaching a person how to apply a condom, or how to masturbate or how to apply a penile sheath could amount to indecent assault, particularly if that young person had a severe learning difficulty. The important issue for the health care practitioner is to ensure that their employment contract or job description explicitly sets out their permitted responsibilities and that the parameters within the job description are lawful. So if the job description outlines that a nurse may explain to a disabled person how to apply a condom, the health care practitioner is undertaking this role legitimately, as a teacher. It is important that the health care practitioner is very clear of the legal limitationss placed on their practice.

Indecency is something that the ordinary lay person would consider indecent. Thus, if a nurse was *teaching* a young girl with learning difficulties how to manage menstruation, by advising her how to change her sanitary towels, this would not normally be regarded as an indecent act. Difficulties *could* arise when the health professional tries to teach a patient how to masturbate. Even if a health professional can assure that the teaching is carried out in an appropriate and professional manner, and that he or she did not physically touch the young person, this could give rise to disciplinary action or a charge being brought against that health professional even if there was no intention to cause harm to that person. It is therefore essential that there are clear, written procedures for any form of sexual advice or intervention, which are mindful of the law, and clearly demonstrate the lines of accountability for the health care practitioner. If such procedures are in place, the likelihood of potential abuse and misunderstanding will be minimized.

Abuse and vulnerability

The Government has recently recognized the importance of reducing the risk of abuse in children, young people and vulnerable adults. The White Paper, *Modernising Social Services* (DoH 1998), heralded the government's intention to provide better protection for individuals needing care, support and protection from abuse. This was further demonstrated by the enactment of the Care Standards Act 2000.

In addition, the Government pledged its commitment to provide greater protection to victims and witnesses, and to ensure the implementation of measures proposed in *Speaking Up for Justice* (Home Office). The report concerns the treatment of vulnerable or intimidated witnesses within the criminal justice system. *Speaking Up for Justice* recognizes that there were concerns about the identification and reporting of crime against vulnerable adults living in care. This Report supported recommendations made by the Association of Directors of Social Services (ADSS), health agencies and the police, that a national policy should be developed to protect such vulnerable adults. In consequence, it was agreed that local multiagency codes of practice should also be developed.

The development of the local codes of practice was co-ordinated by each local authority social services department. To support the process, guidance was issued under Section 7 of the Local Authority Social Services Act 1970.

Contraception and the law

The case of *Re R {1987} 2 ALL ER 206* highlighted sensitive issues regarding contraception. This case concerned a 17-year-old young woman with moderate learning difficulties. Although the teenager was able to manage her menstruation, it was felt that she was unable to deal with or make informed choices about her contraception. The court decided that it was in her best interests and appropriate to sterilize her. While the court found it appropriate to intervene in this case regarding contraceptive methods, it had difficulty in addressing some of the rights issues regarding the sexuality of disabled people.

Sex education

Gunn (1989) and Carson (1987) recognize that staff in schools, residential or community settings have an important role in providing sex education, particularly for people with learning difficulties. In 1993, by virtue of the Education Act 1993, sex education became compulsory in all mainstream and special schools. Teaching about AIDS, HIV and sexually transmitted diseases is included in the syllabus. However, a subsequent Education Act 1997 stipulates that: "a) to consider separately (while having regard to the local education authority's statement under section 370) the question of whether sex education should form part of the secular curriculum for the school". These subjects may not always be included within the Science National Curriculum, which may be limited to the biological aspects of human sexual behaviour.

However, since 1993, the governing body of each and every grant maintained, maintained and special school is obliged to keep an up-to-date statement of their sex education policy. Furthermore, the governing body must approve their school's sex education policy and any personal and social health education courses provided. In addition, all parents have the right to inspect the school's curriculum. Difficulties may arise when parents exercise their right to withdraw their daughter or son from all or part of the sex education syllabus, apart from those lessons that form part of the National Curriculum. The Disability Act 2001, which received Royal assent on 11 May 2001, deals with disability discrimination in education both in schools and higher education. However, difficulties may arise when the young person wishes to override their parent's decision to withdraw them from sex education classes and chooses to attend the sex education classes. The young person might be afforded some legal rights under the First Protocol, Article 2 of the Human Rights Act – The Right to Education.

A school nurse recently asked me about a 14-year-old disabled girl who was a wheelchair user but had no apparent learning difficulties. The disabled girl had challenged her parents' decision to withdraw her from sex education classes. The 14-year-old had an IQ of about 100 and felt that she had the same rights as her peers to attend sex education programmes. Her parents felt that such classes 'would do her more harm than good and would not necessarily be in her best interests'. The school nurse, who had been contacted by the 14-year-old, wondered if the girl might apply the Gillick ruling to her own particular circumstances (*Gillick v. West Norfolk and Wisbeck Area Health Authority and another {1985} 3 All ER 402*). The Gillick Principle, as it is frequently described, was a case that concerned the provision of contraceptive advice and treatment for girls under the age of 16 years. Lord Fraser, in a House of Lords precedent case, stated that providing the person was competent, parental consent was not always required for a girl to use contraception under 16 years. This was in spite of the fact that it is an offence for a man to have unlawful sexual intercourse with a girl under 16 (s.6 Sexual Offences Act 1956). If the Gillick Principle is applied to this scenario, should the 14-year-old be allowed to choose whether she attends sex education classes or not? This is clearly an area where governing bodies, parental choice and children's and young people's rights may conflict. Equally, a 16-year-old may change his or her own general practitioner and decide on his or her own medical treatment (The Family Law Reform Act 1969, s8). However, this does not entitle a person between 16 and 18 years to refuse treatment, if it is not in his or her best interests. Both males and females who are 16 years of age may marry with parental consent. Males and females who are 18 years and older may marry without parental consent, 18 being the age of majority in the UK.

Several people in this research reported that they had been excluded from sex education classes, having been told by staff that they would not need such information. One young man advised me that his teacher had said that he would be better off going to the hydrotherapy pool, as the course would be irrelevant to his needs, without seeking his particular views or wishes on the matter.

People with learning difficulties

The terminology used for people with mental handicap or a learning difficulty has changed over the years. The term 'defective' in the Sexual Offences Act 1956 and outlined in the Mental Health Act 1982 (Amendment) Schedule 3 now means 'a state of arrested or incomplete development of mind which includes severe impairment of intelligence and social functioning'.

'Mental disorder' is defined in The Mental Health Act 1983 as 'mental illness, arrested or incomplete development of mind, psychopathic disorder and any other disorder or disability of mind'. *Mental impairment* and *severe mental impairment* are also defined in the Mental Health Act 1983 and were introduced to differentiate between the small group of people with severe learning difficulties who were previously required to remain in a 'psychiatric institution'.

Consent and sexual intercourse

In the United Kingdom (other than in Ireland where the age of consent is 17), men and women over the age of 16 years may have a sexual relationship with a member of the same or opposite sex, without breaking the law. Even if a girl does not have learning difficulties, it is an offence for a man to have sexual intercourse with a girl under the age of 16. A male may be able to prove in his defence that the girl understood what sexual intercourse involved and had agreed to it, or he believed the girl to be older than 16, and thus not be proved guilty. Furthermore, the notion that boys under the age of 14 years are incapable of sexual intercourse was abolished by the Criminal Justice Act 1993. Thus, boys under 14 years may now be guilty of any of the offences involving sexual intercourse.

7 Translating research into practice

In this chapter, I describe how some of the recommendations of this research were translated into practical measures, such as training materials. In 1993, a training video was funded, designed, produced and evaluated[1], and other materials were subsequently produced in 1995. I hope that the lessons learned from producing materials may assist others embarking on a similar project. Producing materials about sexuality and disability can be both time-consuming and raise further ethical considerations.

Introduction

The 30-minute video, entitled *Sexuality and Disability in Spina Bifida and/or Hydrocephalus*, was designed and produced for adults with these disabilities. This was in response to some of the findings from this research. This video is divided into six sections and addresses the following themes:

- Attitudes towards sexuality and disability.
- Body differences (between able-bodied and young adults with disabilities).
- Genetic risks.
- Explanation and management of continence in a physical or sexual relationship.
- Comfortable positions in a physical relationship.
- Pregnancy and birth.

Attitudes towards sexuality and disability

This section on the video showed disabled people taking part in a variety of activities, including the London wheelchair marathon and Sir Jeffrey Tate, an internationally renowned music conductor who has spina bifida, engaged in his work and social activities. The section concluded with young people discussing their own perceptions of friendship, love, relationships and sex (see Appendix 5).

---

[1] Not available commercially.

Body differences

Using visual illustrations, this section briefly described the body differences between the young person who has spina bifida and/or hydrocephalus and the able-bodied person.

Genetic risks

This section described the importance of seeking advice from appropriately trained specialists about planning to have a child.

Explanation and management of continence

A specialist continence advisor described different techniques for minimizing urinary and bowel incontinence/discomfort during sex and while having a physical relationship.

Comfortable positions in a relationship

The same specialist continence advisor offered useful tips for consenting adults who may have wished to have a physical relationship.

Pregnancy and birth

This section briefly described the experiences of one woman's pregnancy and some of her feelings about having a baby.

Thirty-eight disabled adults, carers and professionals evaluated this pilot training video at a training seminar in 1993. Of these, 76% thought the material was suitable for people with this disability. Some delegates thought it might have been more beneficial to focus on one topic only, and some thought continence and sexuality should have been prioritized.

Aims and objectives

The purpose of the training materials was to:

- Design, produce and evaluate a pilot training video in response to the *Sexual Knowledge and Experiences of Young Adults with Spina Bifida and/or Hydrocephalus* study.
- Evaluate the suitability of training materials for adults with SB/HC.
- Facilitate the development of sex education training materials for adults with spina bifida and/or hydrocephalus.

Background

The World Health Organisation has defined health as "*a complete state of mental, social and physical well being and not just the absence of illness or disease*". Is the definition appropriate in its application to the specific sexual needs of disabled people?

There is no uniform definition of Health Education, but it has been described by Abelin *et al.* (1987) as "*any combination of learning expe-*

riences designed to lead to a situation where people know how to attain health, do what they can individually and collectively to maintain health and seek help when needed". Abelin and colleagues recognize that health education embodies self-advocacy, but hope to influence policy-makers to initiate change where it is considered necessary.

Although it is now accepted that disabled people can lead fulfilling, independent lives, some consideration must be given to the disabled person's rights to a sexual identity and independence. Fundamental to this outcome is the empowerment of disabled people to discuss and educate able-bodied people about their specific needs and considerations which may impact on their sexuality. Collaboration between different sectors of society may be required to facilitate a change in attitude towards the sexuality of disabled people.

Traditionally, health education has focused on the individual, empowering and enabling a person to adopt a particular lifestyle, designed to minimize morbidity (and disease). This paradigm, whose traditional values have been founded on the promotional and preventative aspects of health in a 'well' and predominantly able-bodied society, largely ignores the social, environmental, individual and personal issues which may affect disabled people. The notion of autonomy and rationality which is inherent to Health Education philosophy (Byrne 1986) must also be applied to disabled people. In order to influence change, legislative, self-empowerment features of disabled people must be incorporated into social policy reform, sex education and not least provision of appropriate materials for disabled people.

Ethical consideration

On completion of this research, a report of findings and recommendations was circulated to all ethics committees. Simultaneously, a short proposal was submitted, advising and seeking approval to develop the educational components of this study. As disabled adults were to be invited to advise and/or contribute to this training initiative, I thought it prudent to obtain ethical approval. All committees gave permission and welcomed the development of the practical implementation of research findings.

Fifty-five per cent of the original research sample had requested sex education information in video format. As I wished to avoid inviting disabled adults who had contributed to the earlier research for fear of identifying them, I only contacted adults who *represented the views of the research sample* but had not personally provided the original data.

The question of payment was a difficult matter to assess. Clearly I did not wish to abuse disabled people by not offering some honorarium for their contribution. Equally, payment might be interpreted as coercion. The advisory panel (see Acknowledgments) agreed that reasonable expenses should be reimbursed and a gift voucher offered in appreciation of the disabled person's services.

Methodology

Funding

On completion of Part A of this study, I wrote to the following for sponsorship to develop the materials: Department of Health, Health Promotion Authority, the Family Planning Association, ASBAH, SCOPE (formerly the Spastics Society), local Family Health Service Units (FHSUs), various pharmaceutical firms and continence and contraceptive suppliers. Although all replied and expressed enthusiasm about the project, only Boots the Chemist offered a small contribution. I contacted local health education units for practical and financial assistance, again to no avail. Finally, I contacted the director of the Medical Illustration Group of the former Charing Cross and Westminster Medical School, who agreed to fund and assist with the production of the pilot training video. The director envisaged that the pilot video might subsequently be used to support future training initiatives.

Video contents

Although the video attempted to address some of the key findings from the research, I thought it was important to include a section about attitudes towards the sexuality of disabled people. I felt that it was pointless to address subjects such as continence and body differences without first examining society's fundamental difficulty in acknowledging the sexual autonomy of disabled people.

Advisory panel

I co-opted and invited the assistance of an advisory panel. These included consumers, health professionals, a lawyer, medical artists and a psychologist. The panel advised on the content and development of the pilot video. All meetings between the medical illustration department were minuted and circulated to panel members for comment. The disabled representative was particularly constructive in his comments.

Participation by disabled representatives

The video was produced as a pilot for evaluation and to support future training material applications. I avoided involving too may disabled people in the 'pilot' film, as I hoped to coopt their assistance in future training videos. To discuss sexual matters, particularly in front of a camera, requires enormous courage and sensitivity. It was felt that some disabled adults might be concerned if the pilot video was not shown to other disabled people. Ten disabled people were invited to contribute to take part in the video (five men and five women). Four disabled people agreed to contribute (three women and one man). All four people were sent a letter, outlining the aims and objectives of the video, describing the contents, and offering a preliminary interview to discuss the script. A consent form was also included. All four disabled adults were initially seen at home. The script was designed and agreed with the disabled person. The four people were given time to consider the contents before filming was arranged. Two adults were filmed at home, one woman in the medical illustration unit and one woman in a London hospital (with prior permission from the woman, the medical and nursing staff and the hospital chief executive). All adults were invited to pre-view the video and comment on its 'rushes' prior to editing.

Scripts graphics and stock footage
A research assistant and medical artist helped me devise a storyboard and prepared scripts addressing the contents. These were adapted and amended by the advisory panel. The artist prepared illustrations to accompany the 'Attitudes' and 'Body differences' sections of the video, some of which appear in this book (see pp. 26–7). Prior permission to use any pre-recorded materials was obtained from the relevant producers.

Other contributors
In the absence of funding, it was impossible to employ actors to narrate or provide a 'voice over' for some of the qualitative statements used in the 'Attitudes' section. Dr Martin Bax agreed to narrate the text. Dr Richard Morgan, head of an adult clinic for people with SB/HC at Chelsea and Westminster Hospital, provided medical commentary in the 'Genetics' section. A continence specialist and I took part in the interview sequences addressing 'Continence' and 'Comfy positions'. Along with myself, a research assistant and two young men provided additional dialogue. I had hoped to coopt the services of a disabled interviewer but was unsuccessful in my requests.

Production
The research assistant filmed the two adults at home, using a super VHS tape and camcorder. I filmed the young woman in hospital and pre-recorded films were supplied by companies with their approval. The medical illustration department filmed and provided the remaining footage and graphics.

Post production
All materials were edited by a medical technician and myself in the hospital editing suite. The material aimed to provide a compilation tape to promote discussion about sexuality. The video included interviews, graphics and film sequences of different lengths.

Evaluation
A group of young adults with disabilities, professionals and carers were invited to view, evaluate the video and advise on future development of training materials.

Testing and evaluation

After editing the video, a study day was organized to test and evaluate the material. Seventy-five people (consumers, carers, health care specialists) were invited – fifty attended.

Feedback

Thirty-eight people completed questionnaires (twenty-seven females and eleven males). The mean age of delegates who attended the seminar and video-screening was 38.5 years. Seventeen adult/carers completed written evaluations. The remainder were completed by health/allied professionals and other carers. A 5-point rating scale was used to evaluate the video (5=excellent, 0=poor). The video sequences were analysed collectively and individually. Comments regarding graphics, music and future development were offered: 50% thought the materials were excellent (overall), 21% very good, 11% good and 3% of medium quality. While the evaluations welcomed the inclusion of graphics, music and interview sequences, the following comments, recommendations and criticisms were made from the qualitative assessments:

1. Materials should include more participation and narration from disabled people (75%).
2. Interview sequences should be shorter to consider the individual cognitive levels of the target audience (80%).
3. Professionals, particularly those wearing uniform, should be excluded (60%).
4. More graphics should be included (60%).
5. Materials should be more visually explicit (59%).
6. Everybody supported the future development of video materials specifically addressing the sexuality and disability of people with SB/HC (100%).
7. Future video material should specifically address the subject of 'continence' and 'sexuality' and be designed for disabled adults (90%).
8. The video should include a booklet that describes the video contents and provides 'user' guidance.

Further training materials

You, Your Partner and Continence, an Introduction to Sexuality, Disability in Spina Bifida and Hydrocephalus was produced as a training pack in 1993 by Imogen Carlton with my advice (this is detailed in Appendix 4). This included a video, booklet, audiocassette and samples. The materials addressed a variety of topics related to urinary, bowel incontinence and sexuality. This project followed similar methodological guidelines as to those explained in the pilot video. I was unable to obtain core sponsorship to develop this training package. Clearly other materials and sex education programmes were required which would address a wide range of topics relating to the sexuality of both adults and children with SB/HC. These included:

1. Further video material for adults addressing terminology, bodily functions, genetic risks and childbirth.
2. Audio visual materials addressing puberty and adolescence for children.

8 Case histories

Introduction

This chapter briefly examines the experiences of four men and four women who took part in 'in depth' interviews, in addition to completing a structured questionnaire. Information obtained in this way may be richer, and more appropriately reflect the views and feelings of disabled people. In this way, the disabled person can direct the interview at his or her own pace and may feel less constrained and inhibited than the approach often used in formal questionnaires schedules. Furthermore, the young person may only share details of what they want you to know about their lives; in other words control, or expand on, the content of the interview at their discretion. These interviews, in particular, highlighted certain taboos about sexuality and raised issues about some of the sexual concerns and exploitation that some of these young people were exposed to. They also highlighted some dilemmas about decision-making and choices for adults who may or may not have a learning difficulty. While this chapter does not provide definitive answers, it is hoped that the case examples may assist other health professionals working with people who may have encountered similar experiences. In order to preserve and respect client confidentiality, all real names referred to in this chapter have been withheld. In other words, where people are referred to by their *first names*, these are fictitious. Names are used to make the information more personal and meaningful.

Case One: Carl's story[1]

Carl was a 25-year-old man with spina bifida and hydrocephalus who at the time of interview lived in a Residential Unit owned by a Christian Foundation. Carl had never had a sexual relationship. He told the author that he desperately craved for one. Carl was paraplegic, a wheelchair user and incontinent of both faeces and urine. He had a minor learning difficulty and

---

[1] This case is also briefly described in Blackburn (1995).

was dependent on staff to attend to some of his physical needs, such as assisting with bowel washouts, changing incontinence pads when he was incontinent of urine and lifting him in and out of bed. On one occasion, Carl asked one of the members of staff if a prostitute would be permitted to visit and 'service' (provide sex) him at the Centre. Following Carl's request, several moral and professional concerns were quite reasonably raised by the staff, given the request that had been made. This request also led those responsible to ensure that there was clear sexual guidance and policies in place within the Centre. At the time of this interview, the 'Carers' were mainly unqualified care assistants, although two of the staff were registered general nurses. The staff accepted that if Carl had lived at home and not in residential care, he could have made this choice independently without having to ask staff. He could possibly have made arrangements for a prostitute to visit him at home or maybe even arranged to visit a prostitute himself. However, living in a residential unit with others (both staff and other residents), who might reasonably object to such a request, raised some significant dilemmas. The staff were particularly concerned that Carl might not fully understand the implications of his request. They were aware that Carl, as a result of his hydrocephalus, sometimes, although not always, experienced some difficulties with his retentive memory. Furthermore, the Residential Centre staff were particularly concerned that Carl did not understand the significance of the request he was making, the risks that he might be exposed to, such as exposure to sexually transmitted diseases or possible sexual exploitation. Furthermore, even if such a request had been approved, which is unlikely, a precedent might have been established which might require staff to provide for this type of sexual fulfilment *for other* residents, irrespective of their gender or sexual orientation. Finally, this request posed additional difficulties for staff unable to endorse sexual activity within their Christian Foundation. Carl was refused 'on site sexual therapy'. However, he was advised that if he so desired, he could seek 'such services' off premises but would not be able to ask any member of staff to transport him there. He was also advised of the possible risks of such a relationship. It is arguable that the frank and open discussion which arose between Carl and the team helped to defuse a potentially difficult situation, although it did not provide the sexual gratification Carl was seeking as an adult, and within an environment which he had come to regard as 'his own home'. It also helped staff to recognize the sexual needs and frustrations of some of the residents they were caring for, professional accountability and the boundaries and difficulties for staff as well as the disabled person posed by such a request.

Case Two: Tara's story

Tara was a 25-year-old female with spina bifida who still lived at home with her father. She was incontinent of both urine and faeces and was a wheelchair user. Throughout her adult years, Tara's father had regularly assisted in evacuating her bowels and often assisted with manual evacuation of the bowel. Tara's mother had died when Tara was in her teens.

Tara's father sensed that his daughter now derived some sexual pleasure from these intimate care procedures (bowel and urinary management) and was seriously concerned that such assistance could be perceived as abusive. He considered his responsibilities to both his daughter and himself and sought advise from the local Association of Spina Bifida and Hydrocephalus's (ASBAH) disabled living adviser. The disabled living adviser provided counselling support and offered both Tara and her father some practical help and advice about continence management. Tara subsequently attended a continence and independence training programme provided by ASBAH which aimed to enable her to foster greater bowel and urinary independence and minimize the risk of her father being accused of sexual abuse.

Case Three: Michael's story

Michael, at the time of interview, was a 23-year-old man with spina bifida and hydrocephalus. He was a community ambulator; in other words, he could walk with a walking stick and did not use a wheelchair. He had urinary incontinence. He was also HIV positive and had sought counselling and sexual advice from a specialist adult disability service[2]. In particular, he wanted to discuss issues about his childhood as he recollected, with grief, how he had been sexually abused by his stepfather. Michael felt that being sexually abused as a child had 'confused' his sexual orientation and possibly contributed to his homosexual preferences. At the time of interview, Michael was dying from AIDS. Since completing this work, Michael has died. Although he received emotional support and terminal care from a variety of health care specialists, Michael never came to terms with the emotional scars of being sexually abused as a child. On top of this suffering, Michael tried to remain independent and cope with his complex disability until the last few months of his life. In addition, there was the stigma of being rejected by some people on account of his homosexuality.

Case Four: Cynthia's story

Cynthia was a 23-year-old young woman with hydrocephalus but had no bowel or urinary difficulties. She was also a known drug abuser and had given birth to two children. Cynthia had been raped in her teenage years. Social workers questioned her ability to care for her children independently and were concerned that they were neglected when other carers were not present. A Multidisciplinary Child Protection Case Conference was convened by the Local Authority, following the birth of her second child, to discuss the safeguarding measures for Cynthia's children and their specific needs. The professionals who attended the case conference recommended that both of her children's names were placed on the Local

---

[2] Outpatient Clinic for young adults with spina bifida and hydrocephalus, Chelsea and Westminster Hospital.

Authority's child protection register, under the category of *neglect*[3]. It was felt that registration would enable closer supervision and support for the family by health visitors, other nurses, social workers, etc. A care plan was agreed and the core group met regularly with Cynthia and her mother to ensure that she and her family were receiving the appropriate services and support to enable her to care for her children. The children's names were both subsequently removed from the child protection register and Cynthia's own mother took an increasing role in supporting her daughter's care for the children. Cynthia and her mother also subsequently attended independent living training programmes, specializing in the needs of young families.

Case Five: John's story

John, a 23-year-old man with hydrocephalus and spina bifida, was physically abused as a child by his father. He was a wheelchair user and had both bowel and urinary incontinence and minor communication difficulties. As a child, John's physical abuse was not reported to the Local Authority. He subsequently lived in a residential unit for disabled adults but often returned to the care of his family at weekends where it was feared that he might be subjected to further physical abuse by his father. John disclosed to me that he had been physically abused and that this sometimes occurred when he returned home. I stressed to John that he needed support and protection. With his approval, the information was disclosed to the local authority by the residential unit staff. A case-planning meeting was held and closer family supervision and post-abuse counselling were made available. John's father was interviewed by both the police and social services, but John was too frightened to pursue the matter through the courts as he felt he would not be believed. However, he was provided with support and advice from his local social work team.

Case Six: Sarah's story

Sarah was just 18 years at the time of interview. She was paralysed below her waist, although she could feel some sensation below her umbilicus. She had spina bifida and hydrocephalus. Her mother had been killed in a road traffic accident some years previously. Sarah had severe bowel continence difficulties and required twice daily assistance with bowel evacuation. Her father normally emptied her bowels manually. He too had recently questioned his own responsibilities as he sensed Sarah derived some pleasure from the procedure. Although alternative procedures had been considered, Sarah felt this was the only method she 'liked'. Sarah's circumstances were similar to Tara's, although the fundamental difference was that Tara' s father had recognized his vulnerability in managing his daughter's bowel management. In Sarah's case, a disabled living adviser

---

[3] *Working Together to Safeguard Children*, (1999) Department of Health.

had to draw both Sarah's and her father's attention to their vulnerability in permitting such a procedure to continue.

Case Seven: Jim's story

Jim was 24-years-old and had spina bifida and was a wheelchair user. When he was twenty-one, he had had a sexual relationship with an able-bodied woman. She was five months pregnant and expecting Jim's twins when she was assaulted and beaten to death by an able-bodied man. Jim was understandably very distressed by this event. He subsequently resigned from his job and has been unable to engage in any other sexual or non-sexual relationship with a woman since this traumatic event. He also felt a sense of repugnance as well as personal violation in relation to his own sexuality as a result of the traumatic loss of his partner in such tragic circumstances as well as losing his unborn children.

Case Eight: Lesley's story

Lesley, aged 17, had spina bifida. She could walk using walking sticks. She attended hospital complaining of amenorrhoea and a recent episode of painful bleeding. An ultra sound scan confirmed that she was about 11-12 weeks pregnant. She claimed the father of the baby was a patient she had made love to in a near-by park whilst both were in-patients, during a previous hospital admission. The couple had moved into a flat together following their discharge from hospital. Both were initially happy about the pregnancy and were planning to remain together. However, Lesley claimed that the putative father had a history of violence and as the pregnancy advanced, she decided that she did not wish to remain together after the birth of the baby and planned to leave him. Lesley was eventually discharged from hospital and later had another ultra sound scan to confirm the pregnancy, following her recent threatened abortion. During her hospital visits, she spoke to medical staff and health advisors in the clinic she attended. The health care staff felt that Lesley was aware of the enormous responsibilities she was about to undertake in having a child. They suggested a case planning meeting with Lesley to discuss how the pregnancy should be managed, and support measures that she would require to enable her to care for her child following the birth. Social Services attended this meeting. They also agreed to discuss the domestic violence difficulties that were occurring at home and the risk this could pose to both Lesley and her unborn child.

The above scenarios highlight many issues regarding ethics, and the recognition that some disabled people may need appropriate and life-long protection from sexual exploitation and harm as well as specific guidance about sex.

Overall conclusion

I believe and hope that this work has highlighted the deficiencies in sex education provision for both adults with spina bifida/hydrocephalus and their able-bodied peers. It has demonstrated that the opportunities for having a sexual relationship may only develop for some disabled people later on in adult life, for example after 20 years of age. It also suggests that disabled adults need to preserve both their own dignity and their sexuality and in doing so that they may require access to appropriate information and counselling for life. Education videos appear to be a popular medium for acquiring information about sex. A pilot video addressing several sexual topics was produced by myself and evaluated by disabled adults and professionals. Further productions were recommended and have now been completed in response to the evaluation of the first pilot video.

Many teachers, parents and carers as well as young people have difficulty discussing sexuality in a meaningful and caring manner. In spite of social policy reforms and changes in the law concerning sex education provision in schools, public attitudes about the sexuality of disabled people regrettably have not changed. Many carers and professionals still find difficulty in acknowledging the sexuality of their disabled 'adult children' or clients. Offering training and information to carers and professionals who may be required to advise disabled people may hopefully lead to a much-needed change in society's attitude towards sexuality and disability.

This work has also suggested that sexuality was not limited to penetrative sex. Some people with spina bifida and/or hydrocephalus may never be able to have penetrative sexual intercourse. Other ways of giving and receiving sexual pleasure need to be discussed and explored. Sexuality should be allowed to encompass all that is loving and sensuous (Edser 1988) whilst remaining lawful.

This work has also demonstrated the importance of listening to what disabled people tell us about their feelings and sexual needs. Disabled people have the right to develop confidence in their own lovableness. If disabled people are able to give and receive love, hopefully they will learn to enjoy sexual fulfilment within their own terms, in their own time, regardless of their disability.

Appendix 1

Consent Forms

A

To all young adults

Dear

It would appear that sex education and information for disabled young adults is deficient in both schools and colleges. The Association for Spina Bifida and Hydrocephalus is carrying out a project in North London and Kent which is looking at some of the issues young people face with regard to the 'sex education and knowledge' section of this project into your district. This has been approved by local medical ethics committees and is being sent to young people with the approval of the school.

To obtain a clearer picture we wonder if a counsellor from ASBAH could speak to you at a venue to suit you, to discuss some of these issues related to sex education and information. Any information disclosed will be confidential and in no way will you be personally identified.

Please could you complete the tear-off slip below indicating whether or not you wish to take part in this study and return it to Maddie Blackburn at the above address.

Thank you for your cooperation. We hope that you will feel able to participate in this study, which is aimed at improving the availability of sex education and information for disabled young people.

Yours sincerely

Dr Martin Bax, MD FRCP   Maddie Blackburn
Senior Research Fellow   Research Health Visitor

Counselling
Adviser/Coordinator
Project Supervisor (ASBAH)

I would/would not* be willing to take part in the spina bifida sex education study (*delete as appropriate)

Name ....

Address ....

....

Telephone no ....

Signed ....

B

Young adults in different districts

Dear

We are planning to interview about 100 young disabled adults in North London and Kent between the ages of 16 and 25 years. We are currently doing a study which among other aspects considers young adults' feelings about friendships. We are concerned about the current lack of information given in schools and colleges about sex and personal relationships.

This project has been financed by ASBAH and has been approved by local research ethics committees. I should like to come and talk with .... about some of these feelings, at home or some other place to suit you. If you agree, please could you complete the tear-off slip below and return it in the stamped addressed envelope to me at the above address.

If you would like further information please do not hesitate to contact me.

We do hope that you will feel able to take part in the study which is aimed at improving access to sex education information, particularly for young disabled adults. We would very much appreciate your assistance.

Yours sincerely

Maddie Blackburn
Research Health Visitor

I would/would not* like to take part in the study of sex education and relationships (*delete as appropriate)

Name ....   Telephone number ....
Address ....
....
Date ....
Signed ....

C

For parents of sixth formers

Dear

It would appear that sex education and information about emotional relationships for young adults is deficient, not only in schools and colleges but in general and health education literature. The Association for Spina Bifida and Hydrocephalus (ASBAH) are currently undertaking a research project in North London and Kent which is examining sex education and sexuality considerations for disabled young adults between the ages of 16 and 25 years. This project is based within the Community Paediatric Research Unit which is part of (the former) Charing Cross and Westminster Medical School, London.

ASBAH has received several requests from young adults and their parents/carers for sex education material and information related to young disabled people.

To obtain a clearer picture, we wonder if .... could speak to you to discuss some of these issues. Any information disclosed will be treated confidentially and your son/daughter will not be personally identified.

If you agree for your son/daughter to take part in the study please could you complete the consent slip below and return it in the pre-paid envelope to Ms Maddie Blackburn, Research Health Visitor, at the above address.

Thank you for your cooperation. We do hope you will feel able to contribute to the study, which is aimed at improving sex education, information and literature for disabled young people.

Yours sincerely

Dr Martin Bax, MD FRCP
Senior Research Fellow

Counselling Adviser/Coordinator
Project Supervisor (ASBAH)

Maddie Blackburn
Research Health Visitor

I would/would not* be willing to take part in the ASBAH sex education study (*delete as appropriate)

Name ....
Address ....
Telephone no ....
Signed ....

Appendix 2

**Sexuality questionnaire used for both the pilot study
and master sexuality study**

This interview is divided into two sections and focuses on sex education and the emotional experiences of young adults with spina bifida and/or hydrocephalus. Section A includes general questions on sexual knowledge received at school/college or not at all. Section B is a more explicit interview including questions about emotional responses as well as sexual knowledge and activity. Young adults will be invited to participate in both sections of the interview but will be given the opportunity to participate in Parts A and/or B as felt appropriate. Participants between the age of 16 and 18 will require parental consent to participate in the study[1]. The interviewers appreciate the sensitivity of the subject matter and may seek information from only one of the sections depending on the ability, cooperation and religious beliefs of the subject. Interviewers will use diagrams and charts where appropriate to assist information retrieval as well as assess the interviewee's comprehension of questions[2].

---

[1] This was recommended by some of the research ethics committee due to some concern about those young people with possible learning difficulties
[2] Please note that face-to-face interviews were carried out with the disabled young adults

Section 1

PILOT SEXUALITY INTERVIEW (D)

I	ID	☐
II	MALE/FEMALE	☐
III	D.O.B.	☐
IV	INTERVIEWER	☐
V	DATE OF INTERVIEW	☐
VI	PLACE OF INTERVIEW	☐
VII	DISTRICT	☐
VIII	OCCUPATION	☐
IX	PARENTS' OCCUPATION	☐
X	PART A COMPLETED	☐
XI	PART B COMPLETED	☐

SEXUAL KNOWLEDGE AND ACTIVITY (PILOT)

(Sexual knowledge/education)

(Ring as appropriate)

1(a) Were you given any sex education at school college? Yes   No

1(b) Was this geared towards disabled people?   Yes   No

2. Did your teaching include information about:

    (a) Conception (how babies are made)   Yes   No

    (b) Length of pregnancy   Yes   No

    (c) How babies are born   Yes   No

    (d) Birth control (contraception)   Yes   No

3(a) Please tick the following:

    Where did you learn *most* about sex?

Parents	☐	Social worker	☐
Relations	☐	GP	☐
School lessons	☐	Hospital doctor	☐
College lessons	☐	Day centre staff	☐
Friends	☐	Picked it up	☐
Magazines/books	☐	Other	☐
Videos/films	☐	Don't know	☐
Nurses	☐		

3(b) Have you read any magazines/books relating to sex education?
    (Ring as appropriate)   Yes   No

3(c) Would you like more information about the facts of life?
                 Yes   No
    (Interviewer's probe/explanation)

3(d) Would you like to know more about:
    (ask even if response to 3(c) was 'No')

How the body develops	Yes	No
How babies are made	Yes	No
What happens when a baby is born	Yes	No
How to avoid pregnancy	Yes	No
How to look after babies	Yes	No
How to feed babies	Yes	No
Anything else?	Yes	No

3(e) Where would you like to receive more information about sex education?

Please tick the following:

Parents	☐	Social worker	☐
Relations	☐	GP	☐
School lessons	☐	Hospital doctor	☐
College lessons	☐	Nurse	☐
Friends	☐	Day centre staff	☐
Magazines/books	☐	Other	☐
Videos/films	☐	Don't know	☐

4(a)   Children

Please tick the following:

Would you like to have a child?   Yes   ☐

No   ☐

Don't know   ☐

Not sure if possible   ☐

Already have a child   ☐

4(b)   Do you know if there would be any chance of your child having a similar disability?

Yes   ☐

No   ☐

Don't know   ☐

4(c)   Where did you learn this?

....

4(d)   Does this affect your thoughts about having children?

Yes   ☐

No   ☐

Don't know   ☐

5   Do you have any worries about maintaining long-term relationships?

Yes   ☐

No   ☐

Don't know   ☐

If YES what are these?

....

....

6(a)   Are there any other problems related to sex education
you would like to discuss?

Yes	☐
No	☐
Don't know	☐

6(b)   If YES specify

....

(*Adapted from questionnaires used in Thomas, Bax and Smyth* (1989)*:*
The Health and Social Needs of Young Adults with Physical Disabilities)

Section 2

SEXUALITY INTERVIEW: USER'S NOTES

Master sexuality questionnaire; on completion of the pilot study, the
questionnaire was adapted as follows

SEXUALITY INTERVIEW (D)

i	ID	☐ ☐ ☐
ii	Male/Female	☐
iii	D.O.B.	☐ ☐ ☐ ☐ ☐ ☐
iv	Interviewer	☐
v	Date of interview	☐ ☐ ☐ ☐ ☐ ☐
vi	Place of interview	☐
vii	District	☐ ☐
viii	Occupation	☐
ix	Parents' occupation	☐
x	Spina bifida/spina bifida + hydrocephalus	☐
xi	Religion	☐
xii	Part A completed	☐
xiii	Part B completed	☐

☐ ☐
☐ ☐
☐ ☐

☐

SEXUAL KNOWLEDGE AND ACTIVITY

PART A (Sexual knowledge/education)

(Ring as appropriate)

1(a) Were you given any sex education at school/college?

	YES	NO
	☐	☐

1(b) If YES was this geared towards disabled people?

1 Yes	2 No	3 Can't remember
☐	☐	☐

2   If YES tick the following:

Did your teaching include information about

Conception (how babies are made)	☐	☐	☐
Length of pregnancy	☐	☐	☐
How babies are born	☐	☐	☐
Birth control (contraception)	☐	☐	☐

3(a) Where did you learn MOST about sex? (Tick as appropriate)

Parents	☐	Social worker	☐
Relations	☐	GP	☐
School lessons	☐	Hospital doctor	☐
College lessons	☐	Day centre staff	☐
Friends	☐	Picked it up	☐
Magazines/books	☐	Other	☐
Videos/films	☐	Don't know	☐
Nurses	☐		

3(b) Have you read any magazines/books relating to sex education?

Yes	No	Can't remember
☐	☐	☐

3(c)   Would you like more information about the facts of life?

	YES	NO
(interviewer's probe/explanation)	☐	☐

3(d)   Would you like to know more about:
(ask even if response to 3c was 'NO')

	YES	NO
How the body develops	☐	☐
How babies are made	☐	☐
What happens when a baby is born	☐	☐
How to avoid pregnancy	☐	☐
How to look after babies	☐	☐
How to feed babies	☐	☐
Anything else .... (Specify)	☐	☐

3(e)   Where would you like to receive more
information about sex education?
(tick the following)

Parents	☐	Social worker	☐
Relations	☐	GP	☐
School lessons	☐	Hospital doctor	☐
College lessons	☐	Nurses	☐
Friends	☐	Day centre staff	☐
Magazines/books	☐	Other	☐
Videos/films	☐	Don't know	☐

4(a)   Children
Would you like to have a child?

(tick appropriate box)   ☐ Yes

☐ No

☐ Don't know

☐ Not sure if possible

☐ Already have child

4(b)   Do you know if there would be any
chance of your child having a similar
disability?

Yes No   Don't know
☐   ☐   ☐

4(c)   Where did you learn this?
State...

4(d)   Does this affect your thoughts
about having a child?

Yes No   Don't know
☐   ☐   ☐

5(a)   Do you have any worries about
maintaining long term
relationships?

Yes No   Don't know
☐   ☐   ☐

If YES what are these?
....
....

5(b)   Are there any other problems related to sex education you would
like to discuss? (ring as appropriate)

Yes No   Don't know
☐   ☐   ☐

5(c)   If YES specify
....

5(d)   Do you have a steady boy/girl friend?
(ring as appropriate)   Yes No   Don't know

☐   ☐   ☐

PART B (Emotions and sexual functions)

I am now going to ask some questions about the parts of the body and how you feel about an emotional, physical or sexual relationship.

The young adult may elect not to answer any questions he/she feels are inappropriate.

(Comments for interviewer):
Interviewer where appropriate or necessary will show diagrams or charts to facilitate information retrieval as well as assess the interviewee's comprehension.

F   =   Female-directed questions only
M   =   Male-directed questions only
M/F   =   Both sexes
D/K   =   don't know
N/A   =   not applicable

	Interviewee's Reply		Interviewer Rating	
	YES	NO	YES	NO

6(a) M/F
Have you heard of the word 'puberty'? ☐ ☐ ☐ ☐

6(b) M/F
Do you know what puberty is? ☐ ☐ ☐ ☐

6(c) M/F
Do you know when most people start puberty? (tick appropriate box)

7—10 yrs	11—13 yrs	14—16 yrs	16+ yrs	D/K
☐	☐	☐	☐	☐

6(d) M/F
Do you know when you started puberty?

7—10 yrs	11—13 yrs	14—16 yrs	16+ yrs	D/K
☐	☐	☐	☐	☐

7(a) M/F   Have you heard of the word:
                   period/menstruation?

	YES	NO	YES	NO
	☐	☐	☐	☐

7(b) M/F
Can you explain what it is?
....

7(c) F Have you ever had a period?

	YES	NO	N/A
	☐	☐	☐

7(d) F If yes, when was your first period?

7–10 yrs	11–13 yrs	14–16 yrs	16+ yrs	Never had	N/A
☐	☐	☐	☐	☐	☐

7(e) M/F How often do periods occur?

Monthly	More than mthly	Every 1–2 mth	3–6 mth	Less often
☐	☐	☐	☐	☐

7(f) F How often do **YOUR** periods occur?

Monthly	More than monthly	Every 1–2 mth	3–6 mth	Less often
☐	☐	☐	☐	☐

7(g) M/F Do you know anyone who has had a period?

	YES	NO	Can't remember
	☐	☐	☐

8(a) M/F Have you heard of the word 'virgin'?

	YES	NO	Can't remember
	☐	☐	☐

		Interviewee's Reply		Interviewer Rating	
		YES	NO	YES	NO
8(b) M/F	Do you know what it is?	☐	☐	☐	☐
8(c) M/F	Have you heard the word 'vagina'?	☐	☐	☐	☐
8(d) M/F	Do you know where the vagina is?	☐	☐	☐	☐

(Interviewer refers to chart/diagram)

		YES	NO	YES	NO
9(a) M/F	Do you know where the breasts are?	☐	☐	☐	☐
9(b) M/F	Do you know what the breasts are for?	☐	☐	☐	☐
9(c) M/F	Have you heard the word 'nipple'?	☐	☐	☐	☐
9(d) M/F	Do you know where the nipples are?	☐	☐	☐	☐
9(e) M/F	Do you know what the nipples are for?	☐	☐	☐	☐
10 M/F	Do you know where men and women have body hair?	☐	☐	☐	☐
11(a) M/F	Have you heard the word 'penis'?	☐	☐	☐	☐
11(b) M/F	Do you know where the penis is situated?	☐	☐	☐	☐

		Interviewee's Reply		Interviewer Rating	
		YES	NO	YES	NO
12(a) M/F	Have you heard the word 'erection'?	☐	☐	☐	☐
12(b) M/F	Do you know what an erection is?	☐	☐	☐	☐

		YES	NO	D/K	N/A
12(c) M	Do you ever have erections?	☐	☐	☐	☐

12(d) M   If YES when do these occur?
(Tick as appropriate)

Early morning only	Early morning and other times	D/K	Never	N/A
☐	☐	☐	☐	☐

		Interviewee's Reply		Interviewer Rating	
		YES	NO	YES	NO
13(a) M/F	Have you heard the term 'wet dreams'	☐	☐	☐	☐
13(b) M/F	Do you know what they are?	☐	☐	☐	☐
13(c) M	Do you ever have 'wet dreams'?	☐	☐	☐	☐
14(a) M/F	Have you heard the word 'sperm'?	☐	☐	☐	☐
14(b) M/F	Can you explain what it is/ what it looks like?	☐	☐	☐	☐

....

....

		Interviewee's Reply		Interviewer Rating	
		YES	NO	YES	NO
14(c) M/F	Where does sperm come out of the body?	☐	☐	☐	☐
14(d) M/F	Have you heard the word 'masturbation'?	☐	☐	☐	☐
14(e) M/F	Can you explain what it is?	☐	☐	☐	☐

....
....

		YES	NO
15(a) M/F	Do you ever feel attracted to the opposite sex?	☐	☐
	Do you ever fancy boys/girls?		
15(b) M/F	Do you ever feel attracted to your own sex?	☐	☐
15(c) M/F	Do you ever feel attracted to both sexes?	☐	☐

15(d) M/F   When you feel this attraction what happens?
             (Tick appropriate boxes)

		Opposite sex	Same sex
1)	Blushing/embarrassment/ glowing feeling	☐	☐
2)	Want to touch him/her	☐	☐
3)	Want to smell him/her	☐	☐
4)	Want to kiss him/her	☐	☐
5)	'Tingling' in the body	☐	☐
6)	Other	☐	☐
7)	Nothing	☐	☐
8)	Don't know	☐	☐

16(a) M/F   Have you heard the term   YES   NO

             'sexual intercourse'   ☐   ☐

             If YES what is it?

             ....

             ....

		YES	NO	D/K
16(b) M/F	Have you ever had sexual intercourse?	☐	☐	☐
	(Interviewer may refer to charts/diagrams)			
16(c) M/F	Did you enjoy it?	☐	☐	☐
16(d) M/F	If YES did you feel pain?	☐	☐	☐
16(e) M/F	Do you want to have sexual intercourse (again)?	☐	☐	☐

	YES	NO	D/K

16(f) M/F   Would you know how to get your partner physically excited?   ☐   ☐   ☐

16(g) M/F   If YES how? (Tick as appropriate)

		YES	NO
1)	Looking	☐	☐
2)	Touching	☐	☐
3)	Stroking	☐	☐
4)	Cuddling	☐	☐
5)	Petting	☐	☐
6)	Kissing	☐	☐
7)	Nothing	☐	☐
8)	Other (Specify)	☐	☐

(Interviewee may be offered explanation of terms)

Interviewee's reply

	YES	NO

17(a) M/F   Do you think/did your disability cause any problems when you have/had a physical relationship?   ☐   ☐

17(b) M/F   Do you think there are/would be any problems related to your incontinence and sexual intercourse?   ☐   ☐

If YES tick as appropriate:
Urinating   ☐   ☐

Urine bag leaking   ☐   ☐

Urinary incontinence   ☐   ☐

Catheters:

Suprapubic   ☐   ☐

Indwelling   ☐   ☐

Intermittent   ☐   ☐

Bowels open/
faecal incontinence   ☐   ☐

Others (specify)   ☐   ☐

....

YES   NO

17(c) M/F   Are there any other problems
we have not discussed?   ☐   ☐

17(d) M/F   If YES specify

....

....

Thank you for your co-operation in this study; Ms Maddie Blackburn; Dr Martin Bax; the former Charing Cross and Westminster Medical School (Adapted from questionnaires used in Thomas, Bax and Smyth (1989): *The Health and Social Needs of Young Adults with Physical Disabilities*)

Appendix 3

Coding Frame

Section 1

Coding Frame Sexuality Questionnaire: Quantitative:
Adapted for Qualitative Use

PART A

Box   1–3   ID Code

       4   M = 1 F = 2

      5–10   Date of Birth

      11   Interviewer: Researcher = 1
                                    Counsellor = 2
                                    Doctor = 3
                                    Other = 4

     12–17   Date of interview

      18   1 = Home
                2 = Hospital a
                3 = Other Hospital
                4 = Day Centre
                5 = Residential College
                6 = Other

     19–20   District Code
                1 = Barnet
                2 = Harrow
                3 = Hillingdon
                4 = Hounslow and Spelthorne
                5 = Brent
                6 = Ealing
                7 = Parkside
                8 = Riverside
                9 = Bedford
                10 = Hertfordshire
                11 = EX NW Thames
                21 = Canterbury and Thanet
                22 = Medway
                23 = Maidstone
                24 = Dartford and Gravesham
                25 = South East Kent
                26 = Tunbridge Wells
                27 = EX Kent
                31 = Dorrin Court

32 = Hatchford Park
41 = Other cases
51 = College A
52 = Other colleges for able bodied people

21   1 = Education
2 = Employment
3 = Adult Day Centre
4 = Paid work
5 = Wholly unoccupied
(Michael Hirst classification Social Policy
Research Unit)

22   1 = 1
2 = 2
3 = 3NM
4 = 3M
5 = 4
6 = 5
7 = Student
8 = Housewife

23   SB = 1
SB + HC = 2

24   RC = 1
CE = 2
Muslim = 3
Hindu = 4
Methodist = 5
Other = 6
No religion = 7

25   Completed = 1
Not completed = 2

26   Completed together = 1
Completed separately = 2
Not completed = 3
Not appropriate = 4

27–32   Date of Part B interview if separate from Part A
(Additional Code)

33   Place of Part B interview if different to Part A
(Additional Code) Page 2 Line 1 (cont.)

34   Yes = 1

              No = 2
              Not answered = 9

35–39   Yes = 1
              No = 2
              Can't remember = 3

40–54   (even numbers)
              Parents = 40
              Relations = 42
              School lessons = 44
              College lessons = 46
              Friends = 48
              Magazines/books = 0
              Videos/films = 52
              Nurses = 54

41–53   (odd numbers)
              School worker = 41
              GP = 43
              Hospital doctor = 45
              Day centre staff = 47
              Picked it up = 49
              Other = 51
              Don't know = 53

55   Yes = 1
              No = 2
              Can't remember = 3
              Not answered = 9

56–63   Yes = 1
              Don't know = 3

64   1 = Sex and the disabled
              2 = Giving birth as a disabled person
              3 = Looking after toddlers
              4 = Growth and development related to disability
              5 = Explaining incontinence to one's partner
              6 = Friendship and disability
              7 = Genetic counselling
              8 = Potency and disability

Question 3(e)

65–77   (odd numbers)
66–78   (even numbers)
              Coding as for boxes 40–54

79	Unemployed Yes = 1 No = 2
1	Yes = 1 No = 2 Don't know = 3 Not sure if possible = 4 Already have a child = 5

Question 4 (b)

2	Yes = 1 No = 2 Don't know = 3
3	Doctors = 1 Books = 2 School/college = 3 Genetic counsellor = 4 Other = 5 Not answered = 9

Question 4(d)

4–5	Yes = 1 No = 2 Don't know = 3

Question 5 (a)

6	Discussing disability with boyfriend (1)
7	Losing partner because of disability (1)
8	Partner might leave relationship (1)
9	Yes = 1 No = 2 Don't know = 3
10	Sexual intercourse
11	Kids
12	Other
13	Yes = 1 No = 2 Don't know = 3

SEXUALITY PART B: CODING FRAME

NB   Interviewer's rating throughout this section signifies as to whether the young person:

Understood
Did not understand the terms

Boxes 1–3   Yes = 1
No = 2
Not answered = 9

        4–5   1 = 7–10 year
2 = 11–13 year
3 = 14–16 year
4 = 16+
Don't know

        6   Yes = 1
No = 2

        7   (b) Equivalent to yes/no rating (d) Can't remember = 7

        8   7(c) Yes/not applicable = 9 No codings

        9   Same as for boxes 4–5 **BUT**

                    5 = Never had
6 = Not applicable
7 = Can't remember

        10–11   1 = Monthly
2 = 1 per month
3 = Every 1–2 mth
4 = 3–6 months
5 = Less often

                    Plus box 11

                    6 = Never
7 = N/A

        12–13   Yes = 1
No = 2
Can't remember = 3
Not answered = 9

Boxes	14–32	Yes = 1	No = 2	Not answered = 9

33–35   Yes = 1   No = 2   Not answered = 9

36   1 = Yes
3 = Don't know
4 = N/A
9 = Not answered

37   1 = Early morning only
2 = Early morning + other times
3 = Don't know
4 = Never
5 = N/A
6 = Not answered

38–43   Yes = 1   No = 2   Not answered = 9

44–50   Yes = 1   No = 2   Not answered = 3

51–66   1 if ticked

67–68   Yes = 1   No = 2   Not answered = 9

69   Yes = 1 No = 2 Don't know = 3 Not answered = 9

70   Yes = 1 No = 1 Not answered = 9

71–72   Yes = 1 No = 2 Don't know = 3 Not answered = 9

1   Yes = 1 No = 2 Don't know = 3 Not answered = 9

2–8   1 if ticked

9–10   Code if needed

11–12   Yes = 1   No = 2   Not answered = 9

13–20   1 if ticked

21   Code if used

22   Stoma if ticked

23   Yes = 1   No = 2   Not answered = 9

Box   24   Code if used

       25   Genetics if ticked

Appendix 4

Video Materials

Booklet to accompany video[1]

YOU, YOUR PARTNER AND CONTINENCE

Sexuality, Disability and Continence:
For Adults with Spina Bifida and/or Hydrocephalus, other adults with
Continence Difficulties, Carers and Teachers/Trainers
Permission to reproduce text granted by Imogen Carlton, who
originally produced the video and the text with the assistance of
myself and others listed

FOREWORD

The video[2], booklet, audio cassette and samples form a set of introductory training materials addressing the subjects of Continence, Sexuality and Disability. The materials were designed primarily for adults (over 16) with either spina bifida and/or hydrocephalus and for those with spinal injuries and associated conditions. The materials may be viewed, read or listened to independently, with carers and/or partners or with teachers/trainers.

Practical tips are offered on managing continence for those experiencing difficulty, as well as for those who may be embarking on or already engaged in a sexual relationship. Some techniques and surgical procedures are described. Recent surgical techniques are not described.

Many individuals and organizations have helped with this project[3] without whose valuable assistance the materials could not have been produced. The training materials were produced in response to findings from the research described in this book.

Acknowledgements:
Everyone who took part in the video:
Mr Brian Walsh (narrator), Margaret and Alan Twyford, Kevin Towner, Samantha Lightowler

Producer:
Ms Imogen Carlton

Principal Adviser:
Ms Maddie Blackburn

Advisory Panel:
Dr Martin Bax

---

[1] Not supplied here.
[2] *You, Your Partner and Continence*; Video producer: Imogen Carlton.
[3] Who are listed below.

Dr David Grant
Mr Julian Shah
Ms Jane Williams
Mrs Mary White
Mr John Naudé
Mr Alan Hannah
Mr Brian Walsh

CONTENTS:

How to use the training materials
Continence explained
Urinary catheters and sexual intercourse
Safe sex
Fulfilling sexual needs (for over 16s)
    Section 1
    Section 2
Sexual intercourse: positions
Catheterization
Glossary of terms
Future of continence management

HOW TO USE THE TRAINING MATERIALS

The booklet
This aims to support and develop certain points not discussed in the video. It can be read independently or in association with the video (which is not provided with the book). A list of useful addresses, agencies and further reading are included in Appendix 7.

The video
This lasts for 18 minutes and is divided into several short sections. It may be viewed in its entirety or watched in separate sections/sessions.

Audio cassette
Designed for those who prefer to listen rather than to read. Contains similar information as the booklet and video.

Samples
An attached plastic bag[4] contains some samples which are described in the video, audio tape[5] and booklet. They are not intended for personal use but will give some idea of how the samples appear and feel.

CONTINENCE EXPLAINED

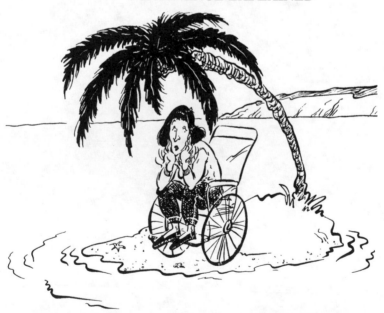

"Incontinence should not make you feel like a social outcast"

---

[4] Not provided here.
[5] Not provided here.

Continence is the process by which you control the disposal of urine and faeces. If you can control this process you are continent, if you have difficulties you are incontinent.

For most people going to the toilet is taken for granted. Most of us recognize when we need to empty our bladder or bowels. Our body will signal when we need to do so.

If you have spina bifida, you are likely to experience some continence difficulties. Your bowels or bladder (or both) will probably be affected. Incontinence should not make you feel a social outcast. There are many ways in which the difficulties of incontinence may be helped, whether or not you are in a sexual relationship.

URINARY CATHETERS AND SEXUAL INTERCOURSE

There are two types of catheterization – intermittent and indwelling.

Intermittent catheterization
If you use intermittent catheterization you should empty your bladder before making love. It is important to do this as hygienically as possible to avoid infection. (Although intermittent catheterization is not a sterile procedure, care should be taken to ensure that a meticulously clean method is used.)

Sample A shows a catheter which may be used for intermittent catheterization.

Indwelling catheterization
If you use this type of catheter, which drains continuously into a urine bag, it is not necessary to remove it for 'love making'. If, however, you do choose to remove the catheter before making love, recatheterize after 'love making' (i.e. having penetrative sex).

Before making love, try to ensure that you have carefully taped the catheter securely to one side (usually your leg) using some adhesive tape.

Sample B shows an indwelling catheter.

Penile appliances
Some men wear a penile urinal sheath.

There are a large range of penile urinal sheaths available to suit most men. Sample C shows one type.

SAFE SEX

Before making love (penetrative sex) you might wish to remove your penile urinal sheath in order to place a condom on to your erect penis. If you are unable to have an erection or have penetrative sex, go to the section on "fulfilling sexual needs" given later in the Appendix for further information. It would be advisable to discuss these issues with your adult urologist or a counsellor.

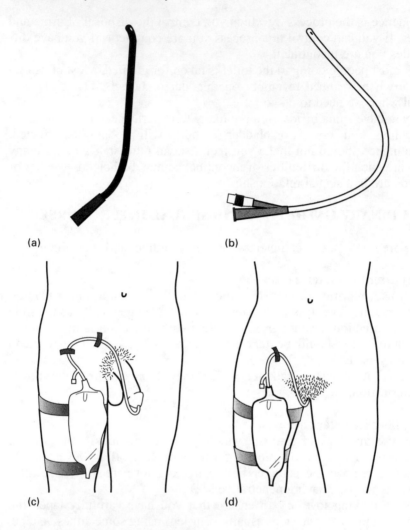

(a)

(b)

(c)

(d)

Figure A4.2 Types of catheters

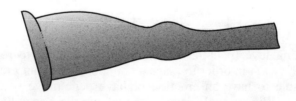

Figure A4.3 A penile sheath

Wearing a condom helps to avoid unwanted pregnancy and infections. If you are unsure or have difficulty in putting on your condom, ask your local Family Planning Clinic or disabled living adviser for advice.

The diagrams below show the different stages of how to put a condom onto the penis.

If you are aware of any allergy or reaction to Latex[6] products, please seek advice from your medical specialist (family doctor or urologist).

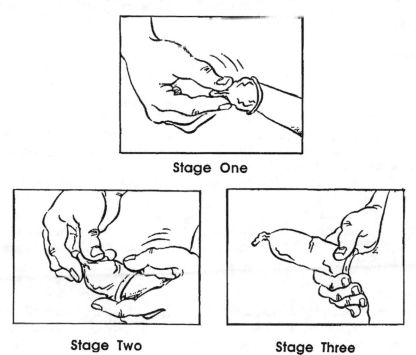

Stage One

Stage Two   **Stage Three**

Figure A4.4 Fitting a condom

FULFILLING SEXUAL NEEDS (FOR OVER 16s)
SECTION 1

If you have spina bifida and/or hydrocephalus you may, although not necessarily, find certain aspects of love making difficult. Sexual expression is not limited to intercourse. There are all sorts of other ways of expressing affection: talking, kissing, hugging, stroking, mutual masturbation and oral sex. These are just some of the ways that both you and your partner can give and receive pleasure from each other.

---

[6] In the USA, in particular, in the early 1990s, several cases of anaphylaxis to latex products were reported in the scientific literature.

Some thought, time and preparation spent discussing sexuality and continence with your partner may help overcome some of the initial embarrassment people sometimes feel at the beginning of a sexual relationship.

SECTION 2

Some people with spina bifida may not feel any sensation in the lower part of their body, particularly around the penis and vagina. Some men are unable to have erections.

Women

Women with spina bifida are able to become pregnant and have a baby. Some women may not feel any sensation around the groin, the vagina or the clitoris and may be unable to experience an orgasm. Sometimes natural vaginal secretions do not occur in this part of the body. It may be helpful to apply some unperfumed lubricant such as KY Jelly to the vagina before making love, to moisten the area, particularly if you experience little or no sensation in and around the groin. The extra lubricant may also prevent discomfort for those who *do* feel sensation, when the penis is placed in the vagina.

Exploring other areas of the body can be just as exciting and may produce an orgasm, for example you may like to try stroking or caressing your partner's breasts or nipples, or massaging their neck, spine, thighs, kissing their face, sucking their ears.

Men

Some men with spina bifida and/or hydrocephalus, although not all, are unable to feel sensation in the lower part of their body or have erections. The penis may not harden and stiffen when the man is sexually aroused.

If you are unable to have an erection or release sperm from your penis, your urologist may recommend giving an injection which will artificially create and sustain an erection for a short period. This does not hurt and usually works!

There are also a variety of other appliances, treatments and operations available to help you have erections. Your urologist or a specialist counsellor should be able to advise you about some, or all of these methods.

SEXUAL INTERCOURSE: POSITIONS

Making love may be difficult for people with disabilities, particularly if both partners are physically disabled. Try to find a position that suits both you and your partner. Try several positions before you find a comfortable one, particularly if either of you have a urinary catheter in place. Lying on top of your partner may be difficult for love making, particularly if one or both partners has spina bifida.

It is *not* necessary to remove your urinary catheter before making love, although many people do! The catheter, for both men and women may be taped to the side of the leg before intercourse (see Figure A4.2c, d). Some people wear absorbent pads and there are many types available (not shown here). If you are worried about any leakage occurring after removing your absorbent pad, you may like to place an absorbent towel underneath the area where you are going to make love.

A little thought, time, preparation and discussion about sexuality and continence with your partner as well as with a doctor or counsellor may help overcome some of the initial embarrassment and difficulty people sometimes feel at the beginning of a sexual relationship.

GLOSSARY OF TERMS

1. Clitoris – a sensitive tissue in front of the urethra of a woman. A woman can become sexually excited when this part of the body is touched either by her partner or herself.
2. Ejaculation – release of sperm from the penis.
3. Erection – stiffening and enlargement of the penis.
4. Masturbation – exciting yourself or your partner sexually. Usually by rubbing your own or your partner's genitals or other parts of the body, e.g. breasts, thighs. It is acceptable to do this as long as it is performed in private – and *not* in a public place.
5. Orgasm – a period of physical release that gives sexual pleasure to most but not necessarily all people.
6. Penetration – in a heterosexual relationship, this usually means inserting the penis into the vagina.
7. Sexual Intercourse – moving a stiff and enlarged penis into the genitals, e.g. vagina.

Further information about planning a family and contraception may be obtained from the following:

- your family doctor
- your local family planning association clinic
- your local Brook Advisory Centre
- your adult health care specialists
- your urologist.

Manual expression
This method should be avoided and only used if advised by your urologist.

Urinary diversion
A urinary diversion operation enables urine to be disposed of through a small opening through your abdominal wall. The opening on the abdomen is called a stoma. The urine is collected in a bag which is attached to the stoma. The bag needs to be changed regularly.

Bag covers
Some people may prefer to cover their bag. You can make one. Some types may be available on prescription (Figure A4.4).

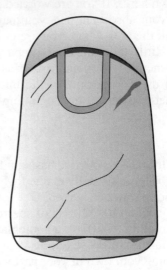

Figure A4.4 Urinary bag cover

Small stoma bags
These are ideal to wear for a short period of time. This makes them suitable for use during love making (see Figure A4.5).

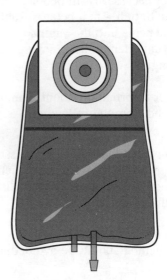

Figure A4.5 Small stoma bag

Bowel management
A healthy diet and regular use of the toilet (at no less than 3–4 hourly intervals) will help you to open your bowels, although you may also require the additional help of laxatives and suppositories.

Hygiene
Regular washing, daily bathing or showering are essential to prevent unpleasant odours. If you worry about unpleasant odours there are deodorant drops and sprays available from chemists. As some people may be allergic to them, choose a type which suits both you and your partner. Care should be taken to use only a small amount as some deodorants and drops are very strong.

Clothing
There are many items of attractive loose fitting underwear available.

FUTURE OF CONTINENCE MANAGEMENT

Urine
Assessment of bladder and kidney function are essential before you consider one of the more recent operations which are now available. Your urologist will be happy to discuss some of these new techniques with you. If you are not already in regular contact with a urologist it would be wise to ask your general practitioner to refer you to one.

The video and supporting materials only describes some ways of managing continence. The standard of urological care and management has improved considerably over the last few years. Surgical procedures have been developed to help you store enough urine and empty your bladder at a more socially convenient time.

Bowels
When diet and regular use of the toilet prove to be inadequate, some people may benefit from the use of laxatives and medications. If self-evacuation is still not possible, some people may benefit from using bowel washouts.

Your urologist or your local continence adviser will be able to advise you of the most suitable ways of managing your bowels. If you would like further information about any aspect of continence management, please contact your adult urologist and/or local continence adviser. Ask your general practitioner or local hospital for details. The Association for Spina Bifida and/or Hydrocephalus (ASBAH) also provide a continence advisory service (their address is in Appendix 7) and regularly update their leaflets.

Appendix 5

Young people's definitions of friendship, love, relationship and sex

DEFINITIONS OF FRIENDSHIP, LOVE, RELATIONSHIPS AND SEX

This Appendix gives some of the definitions that the young adults with spina bifida and/or hydrocephalus provided for the terms 'friendship', 'relationship', 'love' and 'sex'. These four terms were mentioned during the interviews (see Chapter 5). The qualitative interview focused on these definitions (please note that sixteen disabled adults and fifteen able-bodied people provided the information). Numbers 1 to 16 relate to the young adults with spina bifida and hydrocephalus, while numbers 17 to 31 relate to the able-bodied young people.

1.
FRIENDSHIP
– trust, caring, helping, fun,
– being able to talk about things

RELATIONSHIP
– trust and care and understanding
– find security, close bond between you and another person
– how you share your thoughts

LOVE
– caring for someone more than anyone else
– wanting to help them in every way you can

SEX
– depends on the couple
– done for self-satisfaction
– others use sex as a different way to love and express love
– joining together, a bond

2.
FRIENDSHIP
– mutual like for one another
– can talk to and respect
– emotional rapport

RELATIONSHIP
– a mutual attraction and sharing of experiences and affection

LOVE
– strong emotional attraction towards someone of opposite sex
– a natural desire for, caring

SEX
– sharing bodies, meaningfully with someone

3.

FRIENDSHIP
– being able to open oneself to another person
– being able to share your life with them

RELATIONSHIP
– someone who understands me and my needs
– sharing my life with that person and being understood

LOVE
Family love: respect for them, and a place for them in your heart
Friends: special, shared

SEX
– not necessarily in a loving relationship personal feelings, relief of sexual gratification

4.

FRIENDSHIP
– a bond between two people irrespective of sex and gender: sharing love and affection

RELATIONSHIP
– could involve sexual experiences
– (same as above) the bond will be stronger than a friendship
– includes fun

LOVE
– genuine feelings of affection, fondness and concern for something, not include sex necessarily

SEX
– sexual intercourse, between a man and a woman

5.

FRIENDSHIP
When a person can relate to one another, whether its the same or opposite sex, and they can share trust, have a laugh together, and like the same things, something in common.

LOVE
When someone can trust and care about someone, and won't run away from problems, etc.

RELATIONSHIP
When two people care, love and want each other. When people can trust

each other, get on well, be there for each other in times of need, have things in common.

A mixture of friendship and love, which are two important factors of a relationship.

SEX
When a man enters a woman and both give each other pleasure and excitement. It's a natural things and a fact of life. The process by which babies are conceived.

6.
FRIENDSHIP
A unity between two or more people who share many experiences together and who confide in each other, and who are willing to help each other in times of difficulties.

LOVE
A very strong feeling for someone which cannot be explained but felt personally, there is no conventional definition apparently.

RELATIONSHIP
Having an affair with someone engaged in sexual intercourse.

SEX
When the penis penetrates the vagina it gives pleasure, which is often exaggerated by peers and the media.

7.
FRIENDSHIP
This is a relationship in which people are able to confide in one another, have fun, and care for one another, but are not emotionally involved with one another.

LOVE
This is a feeling which extends beyond friendship, where two people are attracted to one another, but can also be something which can exist between relations, e.g. brother and sister.

RELATIONSHIP
This is a broad term used to describe the association of one person to one another. It involves two people who can care for one another in a loving way, or used to describe just the connection between them.

SEX
This is used to describe the process by which a man and woman enjoy sexual pleasure, when the man inserts his penis into her vagina.

8.

FRIENDSHIP
Where two or more people are close and are always there for you when you need them, they understand you.

LOVE
When you get a tingling feeling inside and you cannot stop thinking about that boy/girl.

RELATIONSHIP
Where two people are very close to one another, they are friends not lovers.

SEX
When two people first have sexual intercourse, but are just friends, they are just using each other in a way.

9.

FRIENDSHIP
A person or persons that you can talk to and confide in, someone you can trust and express any feelings and fears, etc., that you have, and have open conversations.

LOVE
Something that makes you feel for someone in a deep way. Like you could really care or someone, and have deep feelings for someone, you're either close to or want to be close to.

RELATIONSHIP
Is where two people can be together, and share feelings with each other. They trust and confide in each other, and be able to talk openly about anything.

SEX
Where two people can show each other how much they love each other, in more than just words. Where two people can be intimate and alone.

10.

FRIENDSHIP
Company with other people, enjoying yourself with them, talking.

LOVE
When you have deep feelings for them you want to be with them, and you don't want them to love someone else, want to kiss and get to know them.

RELATIONSHIP
You have a relationship with everybody around you, it's how you feel

about someone and how they feel about you, is usually positive but can be negative.

SEX
Whether your male or female, when people make love.

11.
FRIENDSHIP
Friendship to me is having a friend you can trust and have a laugh with and someone you can confide in, that to me is what a friendship is all about.

LOVE
Love is a very strong word, you can't just fall in and out of love. Love is being involved, and a bit like friendship but much stronger, feeling of being safe with the person you love.

RELATIONSHIP
Being involved with someone.

SEX
Making love, sexual intercourse.

12.
FRIENDSHIP
Having someone there when you need them.
Someone to laugh, talk to and hug.

RELATIONSHIP
One step up from a friendship, person to talk to. Select that individual because of their special qualities. You wish to be with them more, particularly if from opposite sex.

LOVE
Lots of kisses, hugs, sparkly eyes. The way relates to opposite sex, being caring and kind to either sex.

SEX
Making love: showing love and affection to the opposite sex.

13.
FRIENDSHIP
Trust, respect, sharing and love.

LOVE
Two types:
Parental: more intensified, friendly, involved.

Intense: friendship with someone of the opposite sex.

RELATIONSHIP
An association you have with someone. Links with a person, not necessarily of the opposite sex or boyfriend: rapport, understanding.
Negative or positive.

SEX
Physically become involved usually with someone of the opposite sex.
Love interferes with sex, more than sex interferes with love.
Good sex, not always = good love.

14.
FRIENDSHIP
Loyalty, trust, reliability, dependence on people one considers to be close to them.

LOVE
Similar to friendship, although there can be many different kinds of love, you can love your family and friends (maybe subconsciously) but the love you feel for your boyfriend may be much stronger: of a different kind: when you want to spend every minute of the day with that special person.

RELATIONSHIP
A commitment you make to someone you care about, where in a lot of cases a lot of give and take, compromise is needed, as is trust and honesty.

SEX
When two people consider they love each other or care about each other a great deal by having sex, its the closest they can get to one another and the most that they can give their partner physically. Sex should never be done for the sake of doing it, it should always be done because...

15.
FRIENDSHIP
Two people regardless of sex, can express views and disagree on anything, without causing offence.

RELATIONSHIP
Two types:
Strong: loving my girlfriend long term.
Physical affection: relationship which may disappear in essence of partner.

LOVE
Physical and mental affection, partner's behaviour.

SEX
Two people enjoying a relationship sufficiently to desire to make love.

16.
FRIENDSHIP
Qualities such as trust, honesty, respect, communication, enjoyment of each others company, able to relax with one another, able to talk to one another about problems, fears, feelings, emotions, etc.

LOVE
Deep care and affection for a person.

RELATIONSHIP
As friendship.

SEX
As above, but plus sexual attraction, sexual enjoyment and sexual intercourse.

17.
FRIENDSHIP
Between two people, love between friends, irrespective of sex. Someone you can talk to and trust.
In common and share interests.

RELATIONSHIP
More complicated, falls between definition of friendship and love. Someone to spend time.

LOVE
Someone you can trust and rely on. Happy to share experiences. Mutual, reciprocal relationship, may include sex.

SEX
Mutual bonding of partners, making one feel close.

18.
FRIENDSHIP
Two people who enjoy each others company, in a non-sexual manner.

RELATIONSHIP
Boyfriend/girlfriend relationship, going out with a girl/boy on a steady basis.

SEX
A man and woman having intercourse with the penis in the vagina.

LOVE
Strong feelings of attachment for either a girlfriend, family or best friend(s).

19.
FRIENDSHIP
Two people caring for each other.

LOVE
Depends on who you love.
Can extend love to family, friends and boyfriends.

RELATIONSHIP
Corny friendship, someone is there for you, more general.

SEX
Technically when guy penetrates a girl.
Sex is a broad word.

20.
FRIENDSHIP
Caring for someone irrespective of sex, display loyalty.

LOVE
Between two people.

RELATIONSHIP
Can be sexual, can be platonic.

SEX
Gender, or act of intercourse.

21.
FRIENDSHIP
Friend in need is a friend in deed.

LOVE
Someone who really cares, reciprocal.

RELATIONSHIP
Closeness.

SEX
Physical expression of more spiritual contact.

22.
FRIENDSHIP
No idea.

LOVE
Like a special friend.

RELATIONSHIP
Boys, teachers.

SEX
?

23.
FRIENDSHIP
Sharing and being with someone.

RELATIONSHIP
Friendship with more permanence.

LOVE
The real thing.

SEX
Don't know, nothing at the moment.

24.
FRIENDSHIP
Someone you can truly rely on.

LOVE
?

RELATIONSHIP
Someone you can trust and understands you.

SEX
The act of intercourse.

25.
FRIENDSHIP
Talking to people.

LOVE
Being with someone you like? Girl or boy.

RELATIONSHIP
Someone you like.

SEX
Having a baby.

26.
FRIENDSHIP
Feeling of trust and enjoyment of two or more people's company.

LOVE
Several categories: love and sexual inclination, maternal love.
Extreme trust and care.
Normally expressed towards one individual.

RELATIONSHIP
Several meanings, strong feeling that you want to be with someone and love them sexually
Non-sexual relationship – friends/people/family/teachers

SEX
Actual act of love between a man and woman in order to have a child for pleasure.

27.
FRIENDSHIP
Feeling between people, irrespective of gender, trust and feel comfortable with, attracted to not necessarily sexually.

RELATIONSHIP
Define it in many ways, togetherness, emotional, physical, sexual sharing.

LOVE
Waiting to discover feeling of total fulfilment.

SEX
Physical relationship with person(s), not necessarily having intercourse.

28.
?

29.
FRIENDSHIP
Give and take, trust and loyalty can laugh, cry, and not feel embarrassed with, demonstrate feelings.

LOVE
As above, extension of love different types of love:
Love for parents love for partner/boyfriend
Love for friends, display feelings and understanding for each other.

RELATIONSHIP
Different types:
Parents: my mother is the only person who would be prepared to drop everything for me

30.
SEX
Don't know yet love for a partner, someone who is always there when you need them to be there. Someone who wants me and wants me to be with him.

31.
SEX
Physical relationship, includes touching, kissing and may include inter-course.

Hopefully I may find a partner who will not demand intercourse. There are lots of different ways of making love.

Question mark only: signifies no response or not asked

Appendix 6

Relevant Law

Relevant legislation

Sexual Offences Act 1956

- Rape or attempted rape: section one. Non-consensual intercourse, either vaginal or anal, Maximum penalty, life imprisonment for an indictable(liable) offence
- Indecent assault: sections 14 and 15. Against a woman or man. Maximum penalty – 10 years imprisonment
- Buggery: section 12. This includes male, female or bestiality. Depending on the age of the person involved, maximum penalty may be two, five years or even life imprisonment
- Assault with intent to commit buggery: section 16. Maximum penalty – 10 years indictable prison sentence
- Procurement of women by threats: sections 2, 3, 22, 23, 24, 28. By threats, false pretences, procuring a woman under 21 to become a prostitute or have unlawful sexual intercourse in any part of the world, detaining a woman in a brothel. Maximum penalty – two years imprisonment
- Abduction of a woman by force: section 17: for the sake of her property: Maximum penalty – 14 years imprisonment
- Abduction of girl under 16 or under 18 from her parent or guardian: Maximum penalty: indictable, two years imprisonment.
- Sexual Offences Act 1967
- Sexual Offences Act 1993
- Sexual Offences Act 2000

Offences against the Person Act 1861

- Wounding or causing grievous bodily harm with intent; section 18. Maximum penalty: Life imprisonment

Human Rights Act 1998

- Article 2: The right to life
- Article 3: Freedom from torture or inhuman or degrading treatment or punishment
- Article 5: The right to liberty and security of person
- Article 6: The right to a fair trial
- Article 8: The right to respect for privacy and family life
- Article 9: The right to freedom of thought, conscience and religion
- Article 10: The right to freedom of expression
- Article 12: The right to marry and have a family
- Article 14: Prohibition of discrimination.

Case Law relevant to the Human Rights Act

Botta v. Italy (1998) 26 EHHR 241
This concerned a physically disabled person who went to a seaside resort. There were no ramps, washrooms, WCs or access to the beach or sea. The disabled person alleged violations of Articles 3, 5, 6, 13 and 14 but the European Commission did not feel the provisions had been violated.

Kjeldsen, Busk Madsen and Pedersen v. Denmark (1976) 1EHHR 711
Concerning the rights and choices to receive or refuse sex education.

Other laws

Asexual Offences (Amendment) Act 1992
Care Standards Act 2000
Children Act 1989
Criminal Justice Act 1988(a)
Criminal Justice and Court Services Act 2000
Criminal Justice and Police Act 2001
Data Protection Act 1998
Disability Act 2001
Disability Discrimination Act 1995
Education Act 1993
Education Act 1994
Education Act 1996
Education Act 1997
Freedom of Information Act 2000
Health Act 1999
Human Rights Act 1998
Indecency with Children Act 1960
Mental Health Act 1982
Mental Health Act 1983
Public Interest Disclosure Act 1998
Protection of Children Act 1978
Protection of Children Act 1999
Sexual Offences Act 1967
Street Offences Act 1959
Teaching and Higher Education Act 1998

Appendix 7

Useful organizations and addresses

Useful organizations and addresses

The Ann Craft Trust (formerly the National Association for the
Protection from abuse of adults and children with learning difficulties
NAPSAC)
Centre for Social Work
University of Nottingham
University Park
Nottingham NG7 2RD

ASBAH
ASBAH House
42 Park Road
Peterborough PE1 2UQ
Tel. 01733 555988
Fax 01733 555955

British Association for Sexual and Relationship Therapy
BASMT
PO Box 13686
London SW20 9ZH

British Association for the Study and Prevention of Child Abuse and
Neglect
BASPCAN
10 Priory Street
York YO1 6EZ
Tel. 01904 613605

Brook Advisory Service
Central Office
Education and Publications Unit
165 Gray's Inn Road
London WC1X 8UD
Tel. 020 71833 8488

Children's Legal Centre
University of Essex
Wivenhoe Park
Colchester
Essex CO4 3SQ
Tel. 01206 873820

Community Practitioners and Health Visitors Association
40 Bermondsey Street
London SE1 3UD
Tel. 0207 939 7000
Fax 0207 403 2976
www.msfcphva.org

CONSENT
(Sexuality Training for People with Learning Difficulties)
Woodside Road
Abbots Langley
Herts WD5 OHT
Tel. 01923 670 793

Levenes Solicitors
Specialists in Disability, Personal Injury and Family Law
Ashley House 235–239 High Road
London N22 4HF
Tel. 0208 181 7777
Fax 0208 889 6395
Email:info@levenes.co.uk
Minicom 0181 881 6764

Disability Law Service
High Holborn House
52–54 High Holborn
London WC1 2RL
Tel. 020 7831 8031

Enuresis Resource and Information Centre (ERIC)
34 Old School House
Brittania Road
Kingswood
Bristol BS15 8DB
Tel. 0117 960 3060
Fax 0117 960 0401
E-mail:info@eric.org.uk
www.enuresis.org.uk

Family Planning Association (National Office)
2–12 Pentonville Rd
London N1 9FP
Tel. 0207 837 5432

Health Education Authority
Health Promotion Information Centre
HEA Customer Services
Marston Brook Services
PO Box 269
Abingdon
Oxon OX14 4YN
Tel. 01235 465566

Human Rights Task Force
Human Rights Unit
Home Office
Room 1075
50 Queen Anne's Gate
London SW1H 9AT
Tel. 0207 273 2166
Fax 0207 273 2045
Email: humanrightsunit@homeoffice.gsi.gov.uk
www.ippr.org.uk

Institute of Psychosexual Medicine
11 Chandos Street
London W1G 9DR
Tel. 020 7580 0631

Justice
59 Carter Lane
London EC4 V 5AQ
Tel. 0207 329 5100
Fax 0207 329 5055
Email: admin@justice.org.uk
www.justice.org.uk

MENCAP
Royal Society for Mentally Handicapped Children and Adults
National Centre
123 Golden Lane
London EC1 0RT
Tel. 020 7454 0454

People First
Instrument House
207–215 King's Cross Road
London WC1 X 9DB
Tel. 020 7713 640

RELATE
Herbert Gray College
Little Church Street
Rugby CV21 3AP
Warwickshire
Tel. 01788 573 241
(phone or write for details of local offices)

Royal College of Nursing
Specialists in Physical, Learning Disabilities, Sexual Health
20 Cavendish Square
London W1G 0RN
Tel. 020 7409 3333

SCOPE
National Offices
Assessment Centre
16 Fitzroy Square
London W1P 6LP
Tel. 020 7387 9571

SENJIT
Special Education Needs Joint Initiative for Training
University of London
Institute of Education
20 Bedford Way
London WC1H 0AL
Tel. 020 7612 6273

Sexwise
Chief Publicity Office
Department of Health
Room 579 D, Skipton House
80 London Road
London SE1 6LH
Tel. 0800 282930
(Free Helpline for Teenagers)

SPOD (The Association to Aid the Sexual and Personal Relationships of
people with a disability)
286 Camden Road
London N7 OBJ
Tel. 0207 607 8851/2

Terence Higgins Trust
52 Gray's Inn Road
London WC21X 8JU
Tel. 020 7242 1010/020 7831 0330

Young Minds
102–108 Clerkenwell Road
London EC1M 5SA
Tel. 0207 336 8445
Fax 0207 336 8446
E-mail: enquiries@youngminds.org.uk
www.youngminds.org.uk

FURTHER INFORMATION AND READING

Series of Topic Sheets and Continence 2001/2002
Obtainable from:
ASBAH Disabled Living Advisory Service
ASBAH HOUSE
42 Park Road
Peterborough PE1 2UQ
Cambs
www.asbah.demon.co.uk

Brook Advisory Service:
Booklets on Sex: Contraception, From Child to Adult, Making Love,
Having Sex, Health and Infections
(see address above)

Sex for People with Spina Bifida or Cerebral Palsy
obtainable from ASBAH (Address as above)

SPOD
Your Disabled Partner and Sex
Sex for the Severely Disabled
(see address above)

MS: Sexuality and Multiple Sclerosis
by Michael Barrett of the Multiple Sclerosis Society of Canada

Royal College of Nursing: *Issues in Nursing and Health*
Responding to Rape and Sexual Assault (no. 6)
Guidance for Good Nursing Practice 1995.

Safeguards, Strategies and Approaches Relating to the Sexuality of
Children, Adolescents and Adults with Profound and Multiple
Impairments

Department of Learning Difficulties
The University of Nottingham
Floor E, South Block
University Hospital
Nottingham NG7 2UH
Tel. 0115 9249924

Appendix 8

Glossary of terms

Glossary of terms

The following abbreviations are used in the text:

ABC: Able-bodied controls
ASBAH: Association for Spina Bifida and/or Hydrocephalus
CP: Cerebral palsy
CPS: Cocktail Party Syndrome
CSF: Cerebrospinal fluid
HC: Hydrocephalus
K: Kent
NTD: Neural tube defect
NWTR: North West Thames Region
SB: Spina bifida
SB/HC: When spina bifida and/or hydrocephalus are
                 described together

Carers: Refer to both parents and/or professional carers unless particularly specified.

Health care practitioner: Applies to a health care specialist, e.g. continence adviser, paediatrician, etc., who may or may not be a nurse or doctor.

Please note the following applies to people with minor, moderate or severe learning difficulties:

- Physical disability with no mental impairment: IQ > 70.
- Physical disability with minor to moderate mental impairment: IQ 51–70.
- Physical disability with severe mental impairment: IQ < 50.

(Based on the intellectual functioning category of the Pultibeced classification, cited in Thomas *et al.* 1989, see Bibliography.)

References and
Further Reading

References

Abelin, T., Brzenzinski, Z.J., Carstairs, V.D.L. (1987) Health promotion: concepts and principles in measurement in health promotion and protection. World Health Organization, pp. 63–658.

Alderson, P.A. (1992) Did children change or the guidelines? *Bulletin of Medical Ethics,* **80,** 21–8.

Alderson, P.A. (1993) *Children's Consent To Surgery.* Open University, Milton Keynes.

Anderson, E.M., Clark, L. (1982) *Disability in Adolescence.* Methuen, London.

Anderson, E.M., Spain, B. (1977) *The Child with Spina Bifida.* Methuen, London.

Appleton, P.L., Minchom, P.E., Ellis, N.E., Elliott, C.E., Bol, V., Jones, P. (1994) The self concept of young people with spina bifida. *Developmental Medicine and Child Neurology,* **36,** 198–215.

Association of Spina Bifida and Hydrocephalus (1991a) Information sheet: What Is Spina Bifida?

Association of Spina Bifida and Hydrocephalus (1991b) Information sheet: What is Hydrocephalus?

Bannister, C.M. (1991) Current concepts in spina bifida and hydrocephalus. *Clinics in Developmental Medicine,* No. 122. London, MacKeith Press.

Bannister, C.M., Tew, B. (1991) *Current Concepts in Spina Bifida and Hydrocephalus.* MacKeith Press, London.

Barnes, C. (1992) Qualitative research: valuable or irrelevant? *Disability, Handicap and Society,* 7, Chapter 2, pp. 115–25.

Battle, J. (1981) Culture-Free Self-Esteem Inventory. Seattle, WA: Special Child Publications.

Benjamin, M., Curtis, J. (1981) *Ethics in Nursing.* Oxford University Press, Oxford.

Blackburn, M.C. (1993) Sexuality and sex education for people with disabilities. ABC of disability and abuse. Department of Health, Multi Consortia Training Initiative.

Blackburn, M. (1995) Sexuality, disability and abuse: advice for life, not just for kids. *Child Care Health Development,* **21(5),** 351–61.

Blackburn, M.C., Bax, M.C.O. (1992) Sexuality and disability in spina bifida and hydrocephalus; evaluation of a pilot training video. Short report. *European Journal of Paediatric Surgery,* **2** (suppl 1), 39–40.

Blackburn, M.C., Bax, M.O., Stehlow, C.D. (1991) Sexuality and disability. *European Journal of Paediatric Surgery,* **1,** 37.

Blackburn, M.C., Carlton, I., Bax, M.C.O., Grant, D. (1993) You, your partner and continence. *European Journal of Paediatric Surgery,* 3.

Blum, R.W., Resnick, M.D., Nelson, R., Germaine, A. (1991) Family and peer issues among adolescents with spina bifida and cerebral palsy. *Paediatrics.* Aug (2), 280–5.

Borjeson, M.C., Lagergren, J. (1990) Developmental medicine and child neurology. *Life Conditions of Adolescents with Myelomeningocele,* **8,** 698–706.

Borzyskowski, M., Mundy, A.R. (1990) Neuropathic bladder in childhood. *Clinics in Developmental Medicine* 111. MacKeith Press, London.

Brauner, R., Fontoura, M., Rappaport, R. (1991) *Growth and Puberty in Children with Congenital Hydrocephalus: 1,* chapter 12, pp. 193–201.

Brocklehurst, G., Forrest, D., Sharrard, W.J.W., Stark, G. (1976) *Spina Bifida for the Clinician.* William Heinemann Medical Books, London.

Brookman, R.R. (1986) *Adolescent Sexual Health and Related Problems,* chapter 17, pp. 262–71. Addison Wesley, London.

Byrne (1988) Health Education and Health Promotion. WHO.

Carson, D. (ed.) (1987) *The Law and the Sexuality of People with Mental Handicaps.* University of Southampton Law Faculty, Southampton.

Cass, A.S., Bloom, B.A., Luyxenberg, M. (1986) Sexual function in adults with meningomyelocele. *Journal of Urology,* **136,** 425–6.

Castree, B.J., Walker, J.H. (1981) The young adult with spina bifida. *British Medical Journal,* **283,** 1040–42.

Clark, E., Robinson, K.M. (1989) Research awareness, a programme for nurses, midwives and health visitors. Module 6.

Cromer, B.A., Enrile, B., McCoy, K. (1990) Knowledge, attitudes and behavior related to sexuality in adolescents with chronic disability. *Developmental Medicine and Child Neurology,* **30,** 602–10.

Cull, C., Wyke, M.A. (1984) Memory function of children with spina bifida and shunted hydrocephalus. *Development Medicine and Child Neurology,* **26,** 177–83.

Davies, E., Furnham, A. (1986) Body satisfaction in adolescent girls, *British Journal of Medical Psychology,* **59,** 279–87.

DoH (1991a) Working together – definitions of abuse. Department of Health, London.

DoH (1991b) Working together – consultation paper no. 22. Department of Health, London.

DoH (1991c) *The Children Act 1989, Guidance and Regulations.* HMSO, London.

DoH (1998) *Modernising Social Services.* White paper. Department of Health.

DoH (2000) *No secrets: Guidance on developing and implementing multi-agency policies and procedures to protect vulnerable adults from abuse.* Department of Health and Home Office.

DoH (2001) *Reference Guide to Consent for Examination or Treatment.* Department of Health.

Dorner, S. (1977) Sexual interest and activity in adolescents with spina bifida. *Journal of Child Psychology and Psychiatry,* **18,** 229–37.

Dorner, S. (1980) Sexuality and sex education for the handicapped teenager. *Journal of Maternal and Child Health,* **5,** 356–60.

Dorner, S. (1990) Psychological Problems (1), Chapter 10, pp. 96–110.

Taken from Borzyskowski, M., Mundy, A.R (1990) Neuropathic bladder in childhood. *Clinics in Developmental Medicine* 111. Mackieth, London.

Edser, P., Ward, G. (1991) Sexuality, Sex and Spina Bifida: (1), Chapter 13, pp. 207–208 (2) Chapter 13, p. 203. Taken from Bannister, C., Tew, B., (1991) Current concepts in spina bifida and hydrocephalus. *Clinics in Developmental Medicine* No. 122, Mackeith Press. Distributed by Blackwell Scientific, Oxford.

Edser, P. (1988) Loving ourselves, loving others. The importance of forming relationships. *Link*, issue 1919, pp. 8–10.

Elwood, J.M., Elwood, J.H. (1980) *Epidemiology of Anencephalus and Spina Bifida.* Oxford University Press, Oxford.

Erikson, E., (1963) *Childhood and Society.* Paleden.

Erikson, E. (1968) *Identity, Youth and Crisis.* Faber, London.

Forrest, D. (1991) Foreword: in *Current Concepts in Spina Bifida and Hydrocephalus* (eds Bannister, C.M., Tew, B.). MacKeith Press, London.

Freeman, R.D. (1970) Psychiatric problems in adolescents with cerebral palsy. *Developmental Medicine and Child Neurology*, **12**, 64–70.

Freud, A., (1937; 1946), cited in *Childhood and Society.* Paledan.

Frude, N. (1987) *A Guide to SPSS/PC+.* Macmillan, London. Reprinted, 1989.

Furman, L. (1990) Onset of pubertal development in meningomyelocele. Cleveland, USA (unpublished report).

GMC (1998) Seeking patient's consent: the ethical considerations, General Medical Council. www.gmc-uk.org

Giddings, L.S., Wood, P.J. (1998) Revealing sexuality: have nurses' knowledge and attitudes changed? *School of Nursing and Midwifery*, Auckland Institute of Technology.

Grenier, C., Cartwright, D.B. (1986) A psychosocial profile analysis of spina bifida adolescent in Louisiana. Report for the Handicapped Children's Services Program. Department of Health and Human Resources, Baton Rouge, Louisiana.

Gunn, M. (1985) The Law And Mental Handicap – Consent To Treatment. *Mental Handicap*, **13**, 70–2.

Gunn, M., (1989) Sexual abuse and adults with mental handicap: can the law help? p. 62–63 in *Thinking the Unthinkable* (eds Brown, H., Craft, A.). FPA Education Unit, London.

Gunn, M. (1996) (3rd edn) *Sex and the Law: a Guide for Staff Working with People with Learning Difficulties.* Family Planning Association, London.

Haavik, S.F. Menninger, K.A. (1981) *Sexuality, Law and the Developmentally Disabled Person, Legal and Clinical Aspects of Marriage, Parenthood and Sterilization.* Paul H. Brookes, Baltimore, USA.

Hadenius, A.M., Hagberg, B., Hyttnas-Bensch, K., Sjogren, I. (1962) The natural prognosis of infantile hydrocephalus. *Acta Paediatrica*

Scandinavia, **51**, p. 117–123 in Bannister, C.M., Tew, B. (1991) *Current Concepts in Spina Bifida and Hydrocephalus*. London: Mackeith Press.

Hallum, A. (1995) Disability and the transition to adulthood: issues for the disabled child, the family and the pediatrician. *Current Problems in Pediatrics*, **25**, 12–50.

HMSO (1967) *The Plowden Report: Children and their primary schools*. Her Majesty's Stationery Office.

Holter, I.M., Schwartz-Barcott, D. (1993) Action research: What is it? How has it been used and how can it be used in nursing? *Journal of Advanced Nursing*, **18**, 298–304.

Hurley, A., Dorman, C., Laatsch, L., Bell, S., D'Avignon, J., (1990) Cognitive functioning in patients with spina bifida, hydrocephalus and the 'cocktail party syndrome'. *Developmental Neuropsychology*, 6, 151–72.

James, T., Platzer, H. (1999) Ethical considerations in qualitative research with vulnerable groups: exploring lesbians' and gay men's experiences of health care – a personal perspective. *Nurse Ethics*, **6(1)**, 73–81.

Jirovec, M.M. (1989) Research with cognitively impaired older adults: issues of informed consent. *Michigan Nurse*, **62**, 6–15.

Jowett, S. (1982) *Young Disabled People: Their Further Education, Training and Employment*. NFER-Nelson, Windsor, Berks.

Karoly, P. (1988) *Handbook Of Child Health Assessment*. Wiley & Sons, Chichester.

Kennedy, I., Grubb, A. (1998) *Principles of Medical Law: Confidentiality and Medical Records*: para 9.29: p. 503.

Larcher, V.F., Lask, B., McCarthy, J.M. (1997) Paediatrics at the cutting edge: do we need clinical ethics attitudes towards sexuality research committees? *Journal of Medical Ethics*, **23(4)**, 203–4.

Lebedeff, A. (1881) Ueber Die Entstehung der Anencephalie und Spina Bifida Bei Vogein und Menschen. *Virchow's Archiv fur Pathologische Anatomie und Physiologie und fur Klinishe Medizin*, 8, 6, p. 263. (1882) Lehrbruch Des Allgemeinen Patholoische Anatomie, p. 297.

Lenderyou, G. (1993) Sex education: a healthy alliance, primary health care. *Journal of RCN Community Health Nurses*, **3**, 26–7.

Lerner, R.M., Karabenik, S.A. (1974) Physical attractiveness, body attitudes and self concept in late adolescence, *Journal of Youth Adolescence*, **3**, 307–16.

Lord Chancellor (1997) *Who decides? Making decisions on behalf of mentally incapacitated adults*. Stationery Office.

McNeill, P. (1992) *Research Methods (Society Now)*, 2nd edn, pp. 10–12. Routledge, London.

Madge, C., Harrison, C. (1939) *Britain, by Mass Observation*. Harmondsworth, Penguin (Reprinted 1988 by Cresset Library).

Male and Female Teaching Cards (1983) Education Unit, Family Planning Association.

Marchant, R. (1991) Myths and facts about sexual abuse and children with disabilities. *Child Abuse Review*, **5**, 22–4.

Mazur, J.M., Aylward, G.P., Colliver, J., Menelaus, M. (1988) Impaired mental capabilities and hand function in myelomeningocoele patients. *Zeitschrift fur Kinderchirurgie*, **43**, 24–7.

Medical Research Council (1991) The ethical conduct of research on the mentally incapacitated. MRC, London.

Medical Research Council Study Group (1991) Prevention of neural tube defects: results of the medical research council vitamin study. *Lancet*.

Montgomery, J. (1997) *Health Care Law*. Oxford University Press, Oxford.

Moser, C.A., Kalton, G. (1979) *Survey Methods in Social Investigation*. Gower Publishing Company, Aldershot.

Neale, M.D. (1989) *Neale Analysis Of Reading Ability*. NFER-Nelson, Windsor, Berks.

Neinstein, L. (1991) *Adolescent Health Care: a Practical Guide*. Urban and Schwarzenberg, USA.

Offer, D., Ostrov, E., Howard, K.I. (1984) Body Image, Self Perception and Chronic Illness in Adolescence, in *Chronic Illness and Disability in Childhood and Adolescence* (Blum, R.W., ed), pp. 59–73. Grune and Stratton, Orlando, Florida.

Oliver, M. (1990) *The Politics of Disablement*. Macmillan, London.

Oliver, M. (1992) Changing the social relations of research production. *Disability, Handicap and Society*, 7, 2, 101–15.

OPCS (1998) Congenital Malformations Statistics, Notifications England And Wales. Office of Population Censuses and Surveys.

OPCS (2001) Census 2001. Office of Population Censuses and Surveys.

Philip, M., Duckworth, D. (1982) *Children with Disabilities and Their Families. A Review of Research*. NFER Nelson, Windsor, Berks.

Rankin, J., Glinianaia, S., Brown, R., Renwick, M. (2000) The changing prevalence of neural tube defects: a population-based study in the north of England. 1984–96. Northern Congenital Abnormality Survey Steering Group. *Paediatr Perinat Epidemiol* **14**(2), 104–10

Research Awareness: a programme for nurses, midwives and health visitors, Modules 1–12.

Rieve, J. (1989) Sexuality and physically disabled. *Nursing Clinics of North America*, **24**, 1.

Rogers (1988) The survey perspective: research awareness: a programme for nurses, midwives and health visitors, Module 3.

Royal College of Nursing (2000) *Sexual Health and Nursing Practice*, adapted with permission from the Family Planning Association.

Royal College of Physicians (1996) *Guidelines on the practice of ethics committess in medical research involving human subjects*, 3rd edition, London.

Rutter, M., Tizard, J., Whitmore, K. (1970) *Education, Hhealth and Behaviour*. London: Longmann.

Sandler, A.D. *et al.* (1996) Sexual function and erection capability among young men with spina bifida. *Developmental Medicine and Child Neurology*, **38**, 823–9.

Schilder, P. (1935) *The Image and Appearance of the Human Body*, cited in *Spina Bifida for the Clinician*. William Heinemann Medical Books, London.

Shapland, C. (1999) Sexuality issues for youth with disabilities and chronic health conditions. An occasional policy brief of the Institute for Child Health Policy. FL: Gainesville Institute for Child Health Policy.

Sloan, S.L. (1991) Sexual issues in spina bifida. *Spotlight*. June.

Sloan, S.L. (1994) *Sexuality and the Person with Spina Bifida* (eds Leibold, S.R. Henry-Atkinson). Spina Bifida Association of America.

Smithells, D. (1991) Prevention of spina bifida and hydrocephalus. In *Current Concepts in Spina Bifida and Hydrocephalus* (eds Bannister, C.M., Tew, B.). MacKeith Press, London.

Stanley, C. (1991) In Barnes, C. (1992) Qualitative research: valuable or irrelevant? *Disability, Handicap And Society*, **7**, 115–25.

Strax, T.E. (1988) Psychological problems of disabled adolescents and young adults. *Pediatric Annals*, December 17, **12**.

Tew, B. (1973) Spina bifida and hydrocephalus: facts, falacies and future. *Special Education,* **62**, 26–31.

Tew, B. (1979) The 'cocktail party syndrome' in children with hydrocephalus and spina bifida. *British Journal of Disorders of Communication*, **14**, 89–101.

Tew, B. (1991) The effect of spina bifida upon learning and behaviour, in *Current Concepts in Spina Bifida and Hydrocephalis*, (Bannister, C.M., Tew, B., eds) Chapter 10, pp. 158–79.

Thomas, A.P., Smyth, D.P.L. (1988) The social skill difficulties of young adults with physical disabilities. *Child Care, Health and Development*, **14**, 255–64.

Thomas, A.P., Bax, M.C.O., Smyth, D.P.L (1989) *The Health and Social Needs of Young Adults with Physical Disabilities*. MacKeith Press, London.

Thorpe, L., (1989) Informed decision making. *Nursing*, **3**, 16–19.

Turk, V., Brown, H. (1992) Sexual abuse and adults with learning difficulties: preliminary communication of survey results. *Mental Handicap*, **20**, 55–8.

UKCC (1992) United Kingdom Central Council for Nursing, Midwifery and Health Visiting. *Code of Professional Conduct*.

Verhoef, M. *et al.* (2000), The Aspine Study: preliminary results on sex education, relationships and sexual functioning of Dutch adolescents. *European Journal of Pediatric Surgery*, **10** (suppl 1) pp. 53–4.

Von Recklinghausen, E. (1886) Untersuchungen uber die Spina Bifida. *Virchows Archiv fur Pathologische Anatomie und Physiologie und fur Klinische Medezin*, 105.

Warnock Report (1978) *Special Education Needs, Report of the Committee of Enquiry into the Education of Handicapped Children and Adults*. Cmnd 7212. HMSO, London.

Webb, C. (1989) Action research: philosophy, methods and personal experiences. *Journal of Advanced Nursing*, **14**, 403–10.

Wechsler, D. (1984) Wechsler Adult Intelligence Scale Revised. The Psychological Corporation.

Wechsler, D. (1987) WMS-R Wechsler Memory Scale Revised. The Psychological Corporation.

Westcott, H.L. (1993) Abuse of children and adults with disabilities: policy, practice research series. NSPCC, London.

Wilson, P. (1998) Development and mental health: the issue of difference in a typical gender identity development, in *A Stranger in My Own Body* (di Ceglie, D., Freeman, D., et al., eds) Karnac Books.

Wolman, C., Basco, D.E. (1994) Factors influencing self-esteem and self-consciousness in adolescents with spina bifida. *Journal of Adolescent Health*, **15**, 543–8.

Zarb, G. (1992) On the road to Damascus: first steps towards changing the relation of disability research production. *Disability, Handicap and Society*, **7**, 125–39.

Further Reading

Allen, I. (1987) Education in sex and personal relationships. Research Report no. 665, Policy Studies Institute, London.

Bancroft, J. (1989a) *Human Sexuality and Its Problems. Helping People With Sexual Problems*. Churchill Livingston, London.

Bancroft, J. (1989b) *Human Sexuality and Its Problems. Sexual Aspects of Medicine*. Churchill Livingston, London.

Baric, L. (1990) Primary health care and health promotion. *Journal of the Institute of Health Education*, **28**, chapter 1, p. 22–7.

Barnardos (1993) Meeting the personal and sexual relationship needs of children and young adults with a learning disability. Barnardos, London.

Beardshaw, V. (1990) Last on the list: community services for people with disabilities. King's Fund Institute, 3.3.

Bennett, N. (1974) *Research Design: Educational Studies: a Third Level Course Methods of Educational Enquiry Block 2*. The Open University Press, Milton Keynes.

British Medical Association (1984) *Code of Ethics. The Handbook of Medical Ethics*. British Medical Association, London.

Brook Advisory Centres (1988) Not a child anymore. Training Materials.

Brown, H., Craft, A. (1989) Thinking the unthinkable: papers on sexual abuse and people with learning difficulties. FPA Education Unit, London.

Brown, H., Turk, V. (1992) Defining sexual abuse as it affects adults with learning difficulties. *Mental Handicap*, **20**, 44–5.

Burnard, P., Chapman, C.M. (1988) *Professional and Ethical Issues in Nursing*. John Wiley & Sons, Chichester.

Campion, M.J. (1995) *Who's Fit To Be a Parent?* Routledge, London.

Carmi, A., Schneider, S. (1986) *Nursing Law and Ethics.* Springer Verlag, Berlin.

Childline (1990) Reported telephone contacts to charity concerning abuse.

Cleave, G. (2000) The Human Rights Act (1998) – how it will affect child law in England and Wales. *Child Abuse Review*, **9**, 394–402.

Coile, S., (1991) *Disability, Sexuality and Abuse, an Annotated Bibliography* (Sobsey, D., Gray, S.W. et al., eds), Brookes Publishing Co.

Committee of the Council of Europe (1990) Principle 3 cited in the Ethical Conduct of Research on the Mentally Incapacitated.

Cooper, E (1995) The needs of people with a disability. *British Journal of Family Planning*, **21**, 31–32.

Cooper, E., Guillebaud, J. (1999) *Sexuality and Disability; a Guide for Everyday Practise*: Radcliffe Medical Press.

Craft, A. (1992) Sex education for students with learning difficulties: a resource list. Department of Mental Handicap, University of Nottingham Medical School.

Craft, A. (ed.) 1994 *Practice Issues in Sexuality and Learning Disabilities.* Routledge, London.

Craft, A., Stewart, D. (1992) What about us?: Sex education for children with disabilities. Home and School Council, Sheffield.

Craft, A. and Members of the Nottinghamshire SLD Sex Education Project (1991) Living your life: a personal development programme for students with severe learning difficulties. LDA, Cambridge.

Craft, M., Brown, H. (1991) Thinking the unthinkable: papers on sexual abuse and people with learning difficulties. Family Planning Association Education Unit.

Craft, M., Craft, A. (1987) *Mental Handicap and Sexuality; Issues and Perspectives.* D.J. Costello, Tonbridge, Kent.

Craft, M., Craft, A. (1988) *Sex and the Mentally Handicapped; a Guide for Parents and Carers.* Routledge, London; revised.

DoH (1991) Patient consent for examination and treatment circular HC 90:22. Department of Health, London.

DoH (1991) Local research ethics committees. NHS Management Executive HSG 91:5. Department of Health, London.

Diers, M., Leyin, A. (1983) Participatory teaching materials. Clinical psychologists.

Docherty, J. (1986) *Growing Up: a Guide for Children and Parents.* Modus Books, London.

Dyer, C. (1991) Who decides for those who can't? *British Medical Journal*, **302**, 1352–3.

Ethics Forum (1992a) *Quarterly Bulletin of the National Centre for Nursing and Midwifery Ethics*, no. 3.

Ethics Forum (1992b) *Newsletter of the RCN Ethics Forum*, no. 2.

Ethics Forum (1992c) *Legal Awareness in Nursing*, 4, 1–8.

Fairbairn, G. *et al.* (1995) *Sexuality, Learning Difficulties and Doing What's Right*. David Fulton, London.

Fleming, C., Jones, M. (1993) Teenagers, sex and risk taking: National Brook Advisory Centres. *British Medical Journal*, **307**, 444.

Freeman, M.D.A. (1988) *Medicine, Ethics and Law, Current Legal Problems*. Stevens and Sons.

Fry, S.T. (1989) Ethical Issues in providing care to the cognitively impaired patient. *Journal of Advanced Medical–Surgical Nursing*, **1**, 40–7.

Hanke, G.C. (1987) Sexuality of clients with mental retardation/developmental disability. American Speech, Language And Hearing Association.

Hannah, A.I. (1988 rev 92) Confidentiality. Occasional Paper, 2–3. European Centre for Professional Ethics, University of East London.

Hannah, A.I. (1991) Moral responsibility in nursing and midwifery; paper given at the first National Conference in Nursing and Midwifery Ethics.

Havard, J.D.H. (1989) The responsibility of the doctor, *British Medical Journal*, **299**, 503–8.

Hirsch, S.R. (1986) *Consent, Law and the Incompetent Patient Ethics Law and Medicine*: John Harris (ed.) Royal College of Psychiatrists: Gaskell Psychiatry series.

Hoinville, G., Jowell, R., and Associates (1978) *Survey Research Practice*. Heinemann Educational.

Holborn Reading Scale – George Harrapy and Co. Ltd (1984) Pitman Press.

Holmes, J. (1995) Sexuality and disability; the way forward. Report on a conference on 15 February 1995. BILD Publications, Plymouth.

Home Office (2000) Setting the boundaries: reforming the law on sex offences. Horn, D.G., et al. (1985) Distractibility and vocabulary deficits in children with spina bifida and hydrocephalus. *Developmental Medicine and Child Neurology*, **27**, 713–72.

Hunt, G. (1990) Schizophrenia and indeterminacy: the problem of validity. *Theoretical Medicine*, **11**, 61–78.

Illich, I. (1975) *Medical Nemesis: the Expropriation of Health*. Calder and Boyars Ltd, London.

Keith, L. (1994) *Mustn't Grumble; Writings by Disabled Women*. Women's Press.

King's College London (1990) Ethics Committees in the 90s: role and responsibilities. Conference Report.

Law Commission Consultation Paper No. 128 (1993) *Mentally Incapacitated and Decision Making – a New Jurisdiction*. HMSO, London.

McKenna, A. (1990) Healthy eating and examination of children's preferences. *Journal of Institute of Health Education*, **28**, 5–9.

Marchant, R., Page, M. (1992) Bridging the gap: investigating the abuse of children with multiple disabilities. London. *Child Abuse Review*, 1 (3).

Marchant, R., Page, M. (1993) Bridging the gap: child protection work with children with multiple disabilities. NSPCC, London.

Mary Diers and Alan Leyin Participatory Teaching Materials, Clinical Psychologists, 1983.

Masters, W.H., Johnson, V.E. (1966) *Human Sexual Response*. Churchill, London.

Morgagni, J. (1761) *The Seats and Causes of Diseases Investigated by Anatomy*. Translated by William Cooke (1822), p. 23, Longmann, London.

Moodie, P. (1992) The role of local research ethics committees. *British Medical Journal*, **304**, 1129–30.

Moore, B., Wilmott, A. (1974) Data Collection: A Third Level Course, Methods Of Education Enquiry Block 2. The Open University Press. Milton Keynes.

Morris, J., 1996, *Pride against Prejudice: Transforming attitudes to disability*, 3rd edn, Women's Press.

Murrell, G., Huang, C., Ellis, H. (1990) *Research in Medicine: a Guide to Writing a Thesis in the Medical Sciences*. Cambridge University Press, Cambridge.

Muskett, K. (1995) A simple A to Z OD Sex: a guide for young adults with speech and language impairments. AASIC, London.

NHS Management Executive (1991) Local Research Ethics Committees: Health Service Guidelines.

National Curriculum Council (1990) Health Education Council Curriculum Guidance. NCC, York.

National Legal Center Staff (1991) Medical treatment for older persons and persons with disabilities: 1990. *Developments, Issues in Law and Medicine*, **6**, 341–60.

Neuberger, J. (1992) Ethics and health care: the role of research ethics committees in the United Kingdom. King's Fund Institute, London.

Nurenberg Code (1947) Reprinted in Faulder (1985) *Whose Body Is It Anyway?* Virage, London.

Nursing Standard (1992) Nurses may be involved in unethical research. News Feature. *Nursing Standard* 6, No 32:7.

Owen, O.G. (1994) Sex, contraception and disability. *British Journal of Sexual Medicine*, **21**, S1–S4.

Padma, H., Nathan J.G., Hellstrom, W.J. (1997) Treatment of men with erectile dysfunction with trans-urethral alprostadil. Medicated Urethral System for Erection (MUSE) Study group. *New England Journal of Medicine*, **336**, 1–7.

Royal College of Nursing (1992) Briefing sheets Nos 1, 2, 3, 4, 6, 9, 16.

Shakespeare, T. *et al.* (1996) *The Sexual Politics of Disability*. Cassell, London.

Shevlin, M. and McCormick, G. (1997) Exploring Sexuality and disability: walk your talk. Family Planning Association, London.

Schon, D. (1983) *The Reflective Practitioner: How Professionals Think in Action*. Basic Books, New York.

Sex Education Forum (1992) A framework for sex education. National Children's Bureau.

Sex for Young People with Spina Bifida and/or Cerebral Palsy (1983) published by ASBAH in conjunction with SPOD and Spastics Society.

Sobsey, D., Gray, S., Wells, D., Pyper, D., Reimer-Heck, B. (1991) *Disability, Sexuality and Abuse, an Annotated Bibliography*. Brookes Publishing Co.

Socrates, A. Cited in *Family and Medical Quotations* (1968) (Strauss, M.B., Ed.) Little Brown and Company, Boston, USA.

Spice, M.M. (1989) Sexual counselling standards for the spinal cord injured. American Association of Neurosciences.

Spinal Injuries Association (1993a) Sexuality and spinal cord injury: heterosexual men. SIA, London.

Spinal Injuries Association (1993b) Sexuality and spinal cord injury: gay men. SIA, London.

Spinal Injuries Association (1993c) Sexuality and spinal cord injury: lesbian women. SIA, London.

Spinal Injuries Association (1993d) Sexuality and spinal cord injury: heterosexual women. SIA, London.

SPOD leaflets (Sexual Problems of the Disabled). SPOD, London.

SPOD Leaflet No. 7. Sex and your child with a disability.

SPOD Leaflet No. 9. Contraception for people with disabilities.

Stacey, M. (1988) *The Sociology of Health and Healing*. Unwin Hyman, Boston.

Stenager, W.L. (1995) Sexual problems in young patients with Parkinson's disease. *Acta Neurologica Scandinavica*, **91**, 453–5.

Sundram, J.D. (1988) Informed consent for major medical treatment of mentally disabled people. *New England Journal of Medicine*, **318**, 1368–9.

Taylor, G. *et al.* (1998): Family planning for women with learning disabilities. *Nursing Times*, **94(40)**, 60–1.

Tew, B., Lawrence, K. (1973) Mothers, brothers and sisters of patients with spina bifida. *Developmental Medicine and Child Neurology*, **15** (Suppl 29).

The Children Act (1989) *Guidance and Regulations. Children with Disabilities*. Children In Need, Chapter 3, 5.3.2. HMSO, London.

The Children Act (1989) *Guidance and Regulations. Children with Disabilities*. Children In Need, Section 31 HMSO, London.

The Law Commission (1993) *Mentally Incapacitated Adults and Decision Making: a New Jurisdiction*. HMSO, London.

Tones, B.K. (1985) The use and abuse of mass media in health promotion. *Health Education Research* 9–14.

Trower, P., Bryant, B., Argyle, M. (1978) *Social Skills and Mental Health*. Methuen, London.

Tulp, M. (1652) Observationes Medicae. Amsterdam.

Turnball, H.R., Turnball, A.P., Bronicki, G.J., Summers, J.A., Roeder-

Gordon, C. (1989) *Disability and the Family: a Guide to Decisions for Adulthood.* Paul H. Brookes Co., Baltimore, USA.

United Kingdom Central Council for Nursing, Midwifery and Health Visiting (1987) Confidentiality.

United Kingdom Central Council for Nursing, Midwifery and Health Visiting (1989) Exercising Accountability.

United Kingdom Central Council for Nursing, Midwifery and Health Visiting (1989) Informed Decision Making.

Webb, C. (1985a) *Sexuality in Illness and Disability. Sexuality in Nursing and Health.* John Wiley & Sons, Chichester.

Westcott, H.L. (1991) The abuse of disabled children: a review of the literature. *Child Care, Health And Development*, **17**, 243–258.

Westcott, H.L., Clement, M. (1992) NSPCC experience of child abuse in residential care and educational placements: results of a survey. NSPCC, London.

Williams, B. (1972) *Morality, an Introduction to Ethics*. Cambridge University Press, Cambridge.

Index